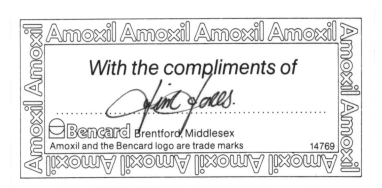

With the compliments of

⊖ Bencard Brentford, Middlesex
Amoxil and the Bencard logo are trade marks   14769

D0229355

COLOUR ATLAS OF
MOUTH, THROAT AND EAR DISORDERS
IN CHILDREN

COLOUR ATLAS OF MOUTH, THROAT AND EAR DISORDERS IN CHILDREN

JOHN BAIN
MD, FRCGP, DCH, DObstRCOG,
Professor of Primary Medical Care,
University of Southampton

PHILIP CARTER
MB, ChB, FRCGP,
General Practitioner, Southampton

RICHARD MORTON
MSc, FRPS, FBPA, AIMBI,
Director of Medical Illustration,
University of Aberdeen

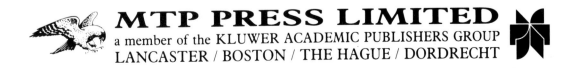

MTP PRESS LIMITED
a member of the KLUWER ACADEMIC PUBLISHERS GROUP
LANCASTER / BOSTON / THE HAGUE / DORDRECHT

Published in the UK and Europe by
MTP Press Limited
Falcon House
Lancaster, England

British Library Cataloguing in Publication Data

Bain, John
  Colour atlas of mouth, throat, and ear disorders
  in children.

  1. Pediatric otolaryngology
  I. Title   II. Carter, Philip
  III. Morton, Richard
  618.92′0951   RF47.C4

  ISBN 0-85200-767-1

Copyright © 1985 J. Bain, P. Carter and
R. Morton

All rights reserved. No part of this publication may
be reproduced, stored in a retrieval system, or
transmitted in any form or by any means,
electronic, mechanical, photocopying, recording or
otherwise, without prior permission from the
publishers.

Typeset by Blackpool Typesetting Services Ltd,
Blackpool, Lancs.
Originated and printed by Cradley Print plc,
Warley, W. Midlands.
Bound by Butler and Tanner, Frome and London.

CONTENTS

ACKNOWLEDGEMENTS

We are indebted to the many children whose mouths, throats and ears illustrate this book. We would particularly like to acknowledge the willing cooperation of the children and their parents who attended for long-term follow-up studies of ear problems and Mrs Helen Thompson and Mrs Margaret McGregor who recruited suitable subjects as part of their work as research assistants.

Many colleagues have given helpful advice and assistance and particular thanks should go to Mr Howard Young, Consultant ENT Surgeon, and Mr William McKerrow, Senior ENT Registrar, Aberdeen Royal Infirmary and Dr Gordon Hickish, General Practitioner, Hampshire.

Finally we would like to thank Mrs Brenda Thomason and Miss Sandra Martin for their painstaking efforts in typing and re-typing the manuscript.

PREFACE

Disorders of the upper respiratory tract and the ear account for almost 50% of all illness in children under 5 years and 30% in children aged 5–12 years. The time taken to examine the mouth, throat and ear in a young child is frequently brief and often no more than a fleeting glimpse can be obtained of the area affected. With this in mind we considered that an atlas of common conditions was required in the literature of childhood diseases.

This atlas includes conditions which lend themselves to illustration and is by no means comprehensive. The photographs were all taken from children presenting in general practice in the United Kingdom and are intended to help students, nurses and doctors recognise the variety of appearances common to children with upper respiratory tract complaints. Illustrations in conventional textbooks tend to show more severe and rare conditions, but we have attempted to provide a range of pictures, including normal appearances, which are representative of conditions seen by those working in primary medical care.

The photographs of throats were taken on Kodachrome 64 film using a Micro Nikkor 55 mm lens and a Nikkormat FTN camera with a Sunpak GX 8R ringflash.

In the case of ear examination, photography through an auriscope provides serious limitations as the pictures obtained give only a narrow angle of view allowing only a small area of the tympanic membrane to be seen at one time. For this reason, the ear photographs were taken using a 4 mm diameter Storz Tele-otoscope. This provides a wide-angle view of the whole eardrum and adjacent external auditory canal. A Nikon FE camera with a 100 mm lens was used and illumination was provided by a high intensity xenon endoscope light source.

The photographs of the mouth and throat were taken by Philip Carter and were from patients in his own practice. The ear photographs came from a variety of practices in Aberdeen and Southampton and were taken by Richard Morton.

PART 1. MOUTH AND
THROAT DISORDERS

1. LOOKING INTO THE MOUTH AND THROAT

Figure 1 It is important to put the child at ease during examination. The approach will depend on the age of the child and the degree of cooperation that can be elicited. In younger children examination of the mouth is best performed with the child sitting on the mother's knee facing the examiner and with the parent restraining the child's head and arms.

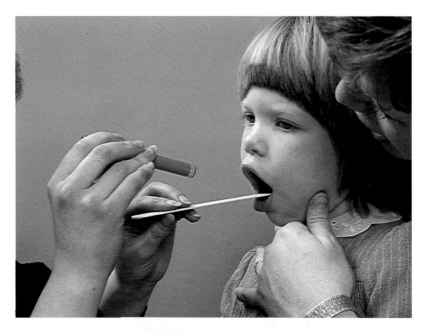

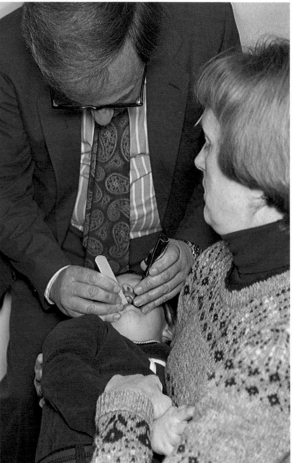

Figure 2 An alternative method particularly suitable with very small children is to have the child lying on the mother's lap allowing the doctor to examine the throat from above.

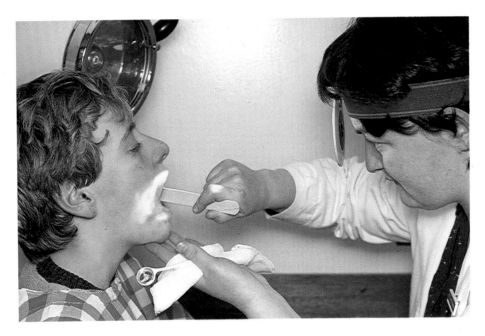

Figure 3 Examination of the mouth is best undertaken with a head mirror and good light source. Preliminary inspection of mouth, tongue, fauces and tonsillar beds is carried out using a tongue depressor.

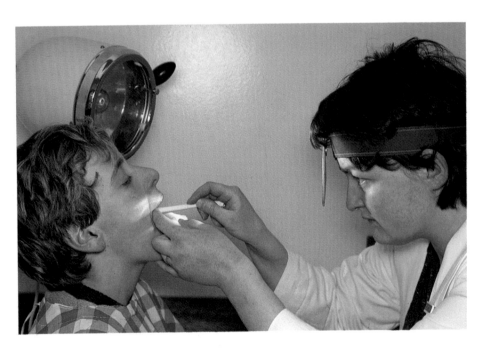

Figure 4 Indirect examination of the pharynx, base of the tongue and larynx with a laryngeal mirror. Requirements are a good light source, head mirror and swab for holding the tongue.

2. THE TONGUE

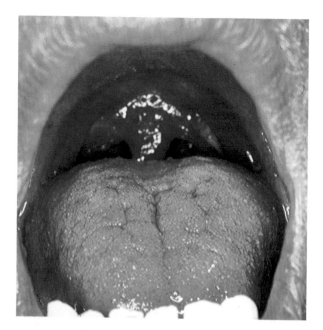

Figure 5 Fissures of the tongue which are a variant of normal.

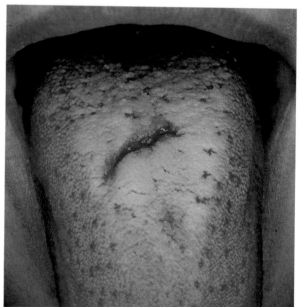

Figure 6 A coated tongue with a deep transverse fissure. The condition occurred spontaneously with no history of injury. It returned to normal without intervention.

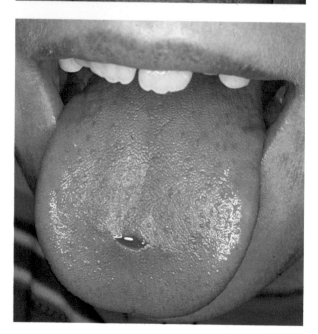

Figure 7 This child fell over his toys and his upper incisors punctured his tongue. Parents can be reassured that a wound of this type will heal within a week without treatment.

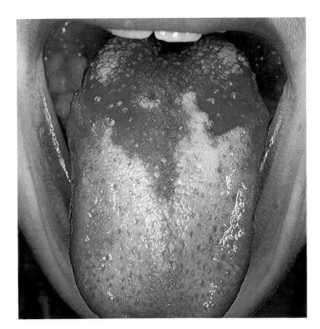

Figure 8 A geographical tongue. This appearance may be alarming to parents who notice it but there are no implications of disease.

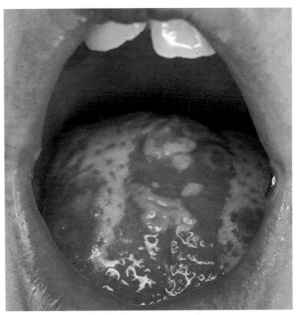

Figure 9 A coated and ulcerated tongue due to herpes simplex infection; also known as trench mouth. The pain is considerable and may require parenteral relief. Ice cubes are often helpful.

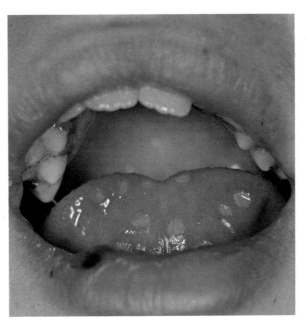

Figure 10 The multiple ulcers of primary herpes simplex. Ice cubes were not enough to relieve the symptoms and the anaesthetic action of Phenol mouth wash gave only brief relief (see also Figure 21).

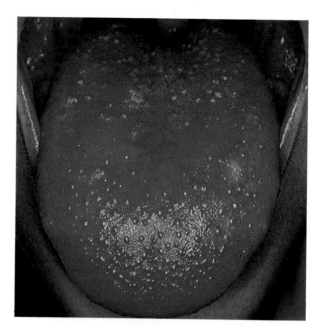

Figure 11 A classical 'red strawberry' tongue, seen here in acute streptococcal scarlet fever.

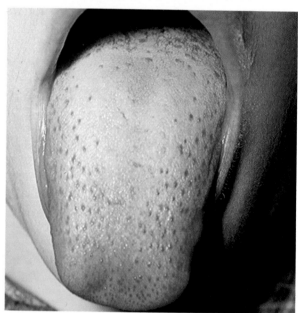

Figure 12 'White strawberry' tongue. This appearance is common in many infections and also compatible with normal health.

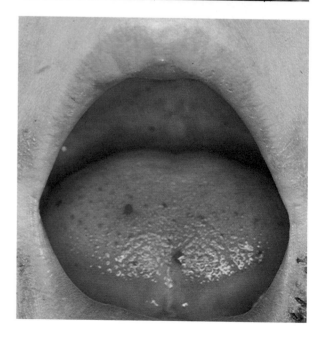

Figure 13 The petechial lesions on this tongue are due to idiopathic thrombocytopenic purpura. This patient's palate is shown in Figure 29. Her parents and doctor had a few anxious days until the diagnosis was confirmed, since acute leukaemia may present with exactly the same picture.

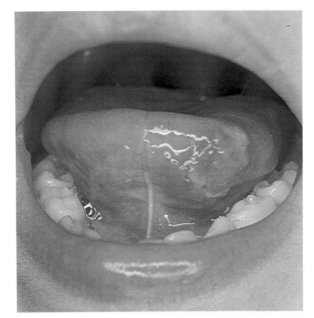

Figures 14, 15 and 16 Hand-foot-and-mouth disease or Toronto spots (after the hospital where it was first described). This is a syndrome caused by strains of enterovirus (*Coxsackie A*). The lesion shown is on the tongue but the buccal mucosa should be inspected as well. Apart from the hands and feet, lesions may also appear on the buttocks. With children in nappies, vesicles, like small flat chickenpox spots, may often be seen.

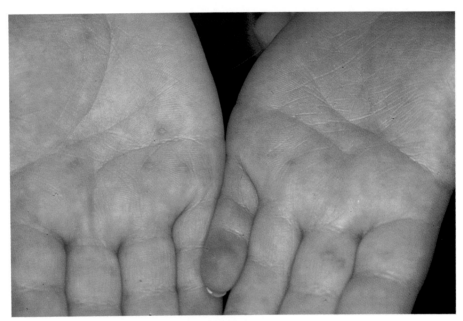

Figure 15

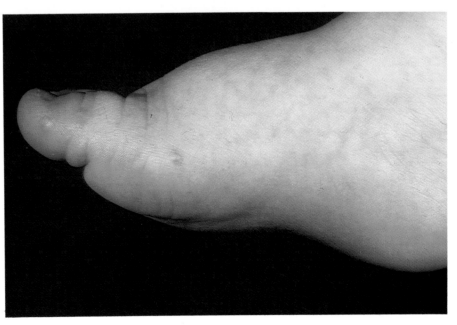

Figure 16

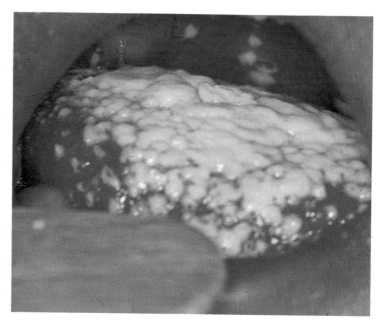

Figure 17 Thrush, a superficial infection by the pathogenic yeast *Candida albicans*. The hyphae of the vegetative phase form characteristic white spots, one or two millimetres across, which may become confluent.

3. THE BUCCAL MUCOUS MEMBRANE

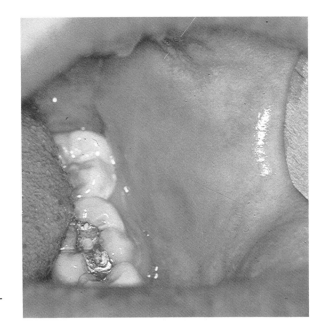

Figure 18 Normal appearance of the mucous membrane.

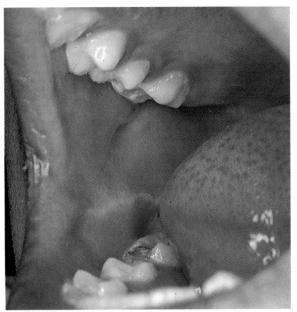

Figure 19 The impression of the molar teeth on the buccal mucous membrane which is a sign of febrile illness, though no more specific than a raised temperature. Often visible as a whitish line it may also be a simple contoured impression with no colour contrast. The whitish lines of the oedematous oral mucosa in fever may also form a ripple pattern inside the cheeks (see Figure 45).

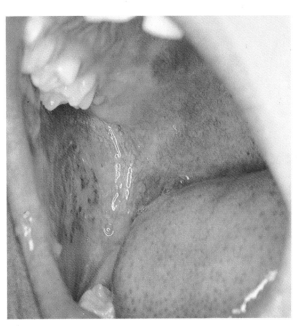

Figure 20 Petechiae due to accidental biting of the cheek.

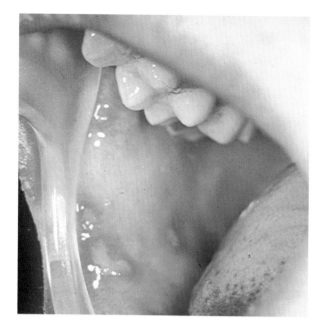

Figure 21 Vesicular eruption of primary herpetic stomatitis (see also Figure 10).

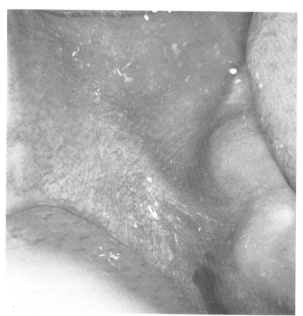

Figures 22 and 23 Koplik's spots in measles.

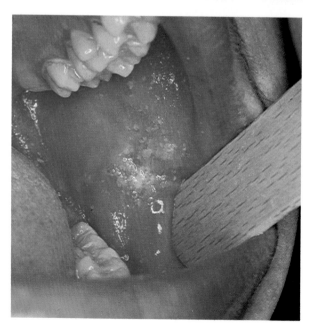

Figure 23

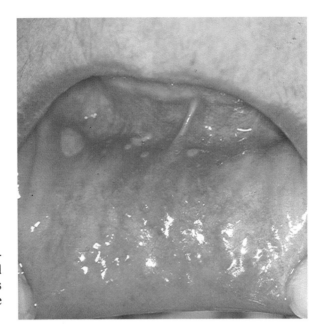

Figure 24 Apthae or aphthous ulcers in the characteristic site in the anterior sulcus. Pain is a noted feature of these unpleasant recurrent ulcers. Relief is given by Triamcinolone in a special dental paste (Adcortyl in Orabase).

4. THE PALATE

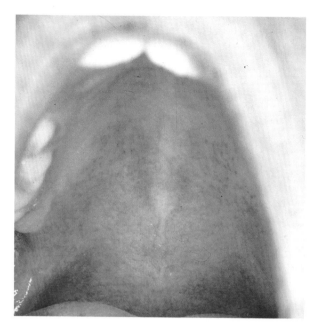

Figure 25 Normal palate showing a slight difference in colour between the soft and hard palate.

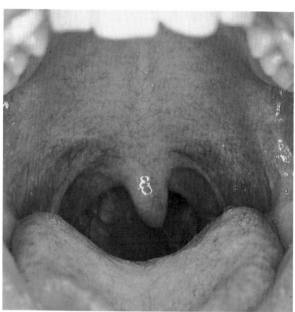

Figure 26 Normal palate and uvula with no colour difference between the hard and soft palate.

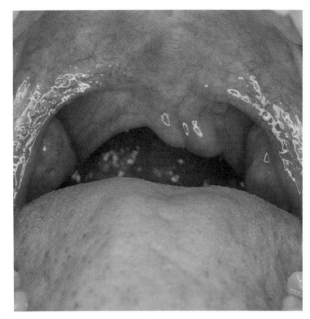

Figure 27 An excellent cosmetic and functional repair of a complete hare-lip and cleft palate. Only the pale scars and double uvula remain.

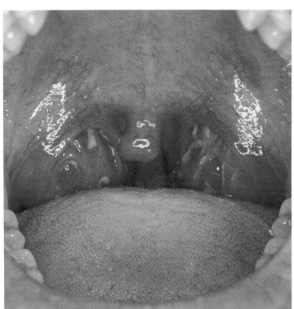

Figure 28 Exudative pharyngitis in a patient with a 'hole in the uvula', a simple variation of cleft palate, or the commoner bifid uvula.

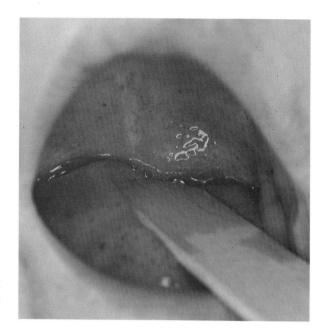

Figure 29 A few petechiae on the palate of a patient with idiopathic thrombocytopenic purpura. This patient's tongue is shown in Figure 13.

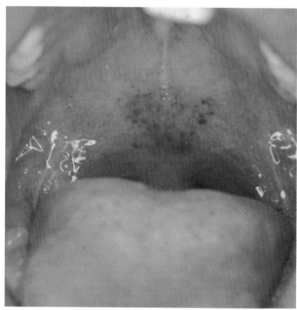

Figure 30 This circumscribed group of petechiae on the soft palate was found during the examination of a child with earache (no signs in the ears). Throat culture was negative for β-*haemolytic streptococci*. He was observed for seven days but no petechiae appeared elsewhere. The palatal group faded in four days.

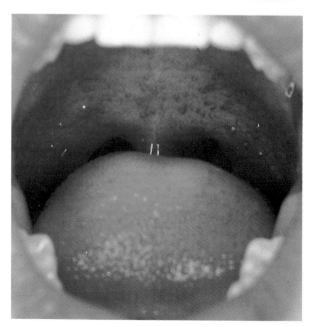

Figure 31 The palatal petechial rash of scarlet fever. Throat culture showed a '3 plus' growth of *Group A* β-*haemolytic streptococci*. The patient was treated with oral penicillin.

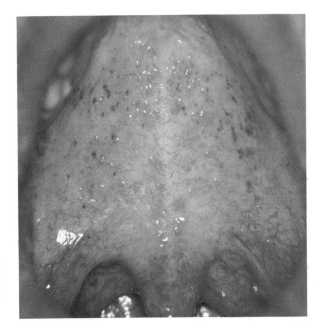

Figure 32 Petechiae which are not in the classical position at the line of the junction of the soft and hard palate. Infectious mononucleosis – same patient as Figure 33.

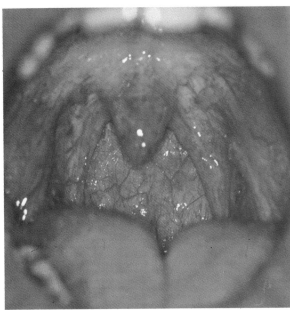

Figure 33 Moderate erythema of the pharynx. The tonsils are small and hidden by the anterior pillars. There is no visible exudate. The blood picture was that of infective mononucleosis. Throat culture was negative for *β-haemolytic streptococcus.*

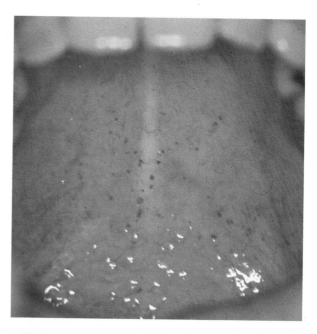

Figures 34 and 35 The age of this patient (16) with petechiae on the palate gave the clue to her diagnosis. She had easily palpable nodes in all four triangles of the neck. Her Paul Bunnell test was positive and she had a Downey lymphocytosis indicating infective mononucleosis.

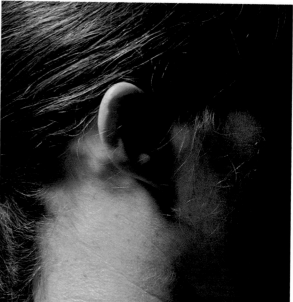

Figure 35

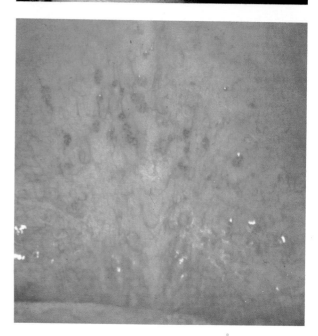

Figure 36 Close-up view of palatal petechiae in a case of infective mononucleosis. As with the cases illustrated in Figures 32 and 34 an additional sign on the posterior soft palate can be seen where the reflections of the flash used to take the picture pick out some six to twelve macules or papules. This appearance is discussed further below.

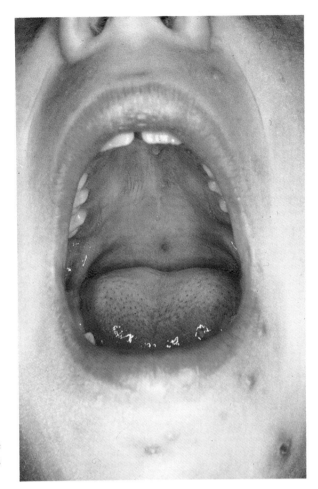

Figure 37 Chickenpox. The central vesicle on the palate is matched by other typical lesions on this patient's face.

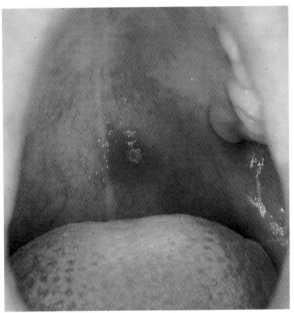

Figure 38 A classic umbilicated chickenpox vesicle with marginal erythema on the soft palate. Dysphagia can be very distressing in chickenpox as the mucosal lesions may also spread through the respiratory and gastrointestinal tract resulting in bleeding from the rectum or, rarely, haemoptysis.

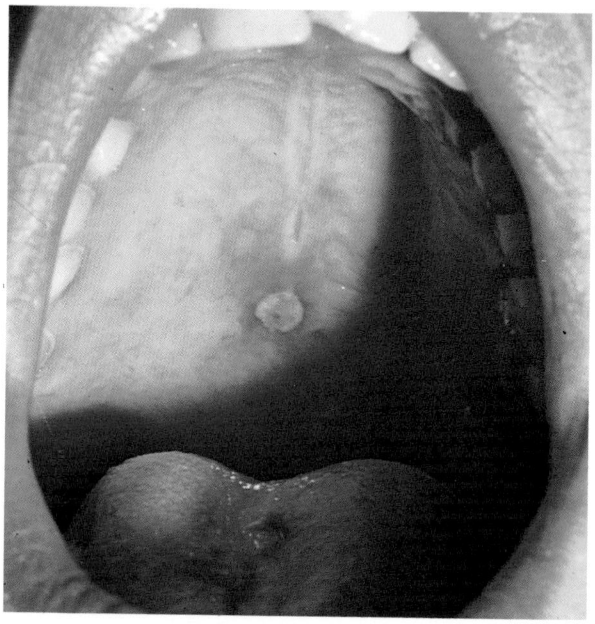

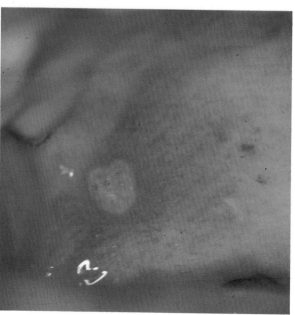

Figure 39 This ulcer was due to a corticosteroid inhaler being used very close to the palate. It cleared up when the use of the inhaler was stopped for a few days and the patient given instruction on its correct use.

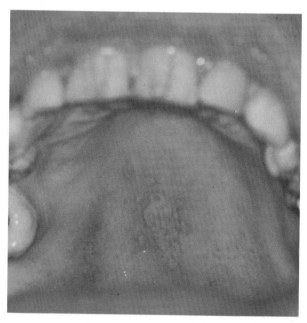

Figure 40 This girl had recurrent 'sore throats' when her herpes simplex recurred on her palate. It was too painful to clean her teeth.

Figure 41 Palatal ulcer with adjacent petechiae. This boy had recurrent attacks since experiencing herpangina at the age of four. He suffered from recurrent pharyngeal ulcers since the original attack, averaging two attacks each year. When tissue culture enabled the agent of herpangina to be isolated it was identified as a *Coxsackie A* virus (usually of group 16 or 22).

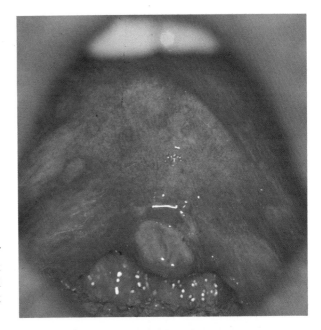

Figure 42 This is more typical of the appearance of herpangina, the large shallow red-rimmed ulcers last only three or four days. They are much less painful than aphthous or herpetic ulcers and the patient is not always aware of them.

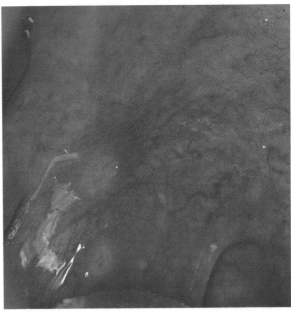

Figure 43 Herpangina ulcers just in front of the anterior pillar of the right tonsil.

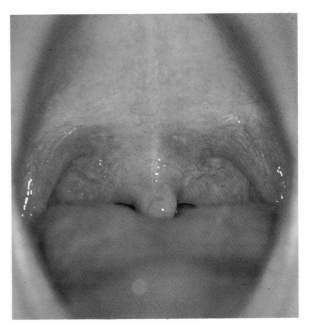

Figure 44 Small herpanginal ulcers confined to the fauces.

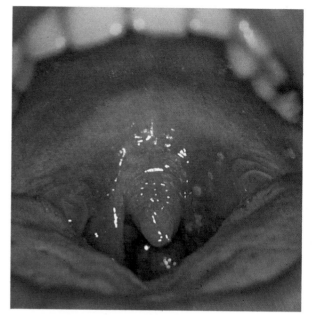

Figure 45 Ulcers together with 'contour lines' of oedema or exudate. This infection was associated with the blood picture of infective mononucleosis.

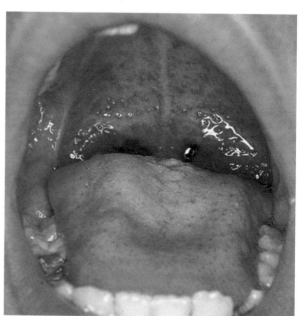

Figure 46 Red papular enanthem of the palate. Attempts at isolation of an infective agent were negative.

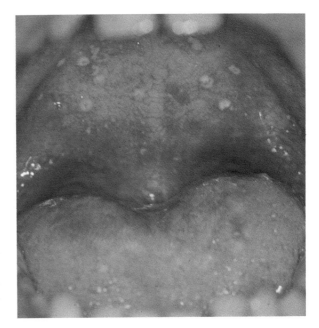

Figures 47 (right) and 48 (below) Steigman's sign. In 1962 Steigman and others (*J. Pediatr.*, **61**, 331) described an outbreak of mild febrile illness in which the palatal and conjunctival lesions were not ulcerative. Their description classifies the lesion as 'lymphonodular' and the whole syndrome as 'acute lymphonodular pharyngitis'.

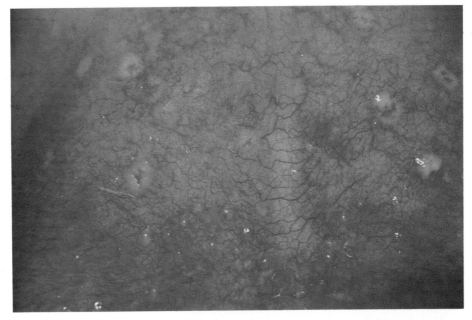

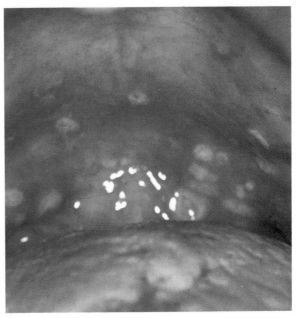

Figure 49 A gross example of Steigman's palatal papules verging on herpangina.

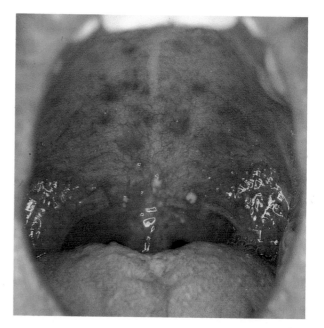

Figure 50 (right)   This eruption appeared six days after a polio vaccination. The throat culture showed only vaccine strains of polio virus suggesting that the eruption, which shows both red and white papules, was due to the polio virus, which is an enterovirus.

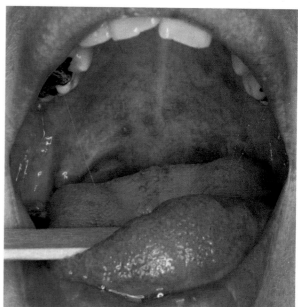

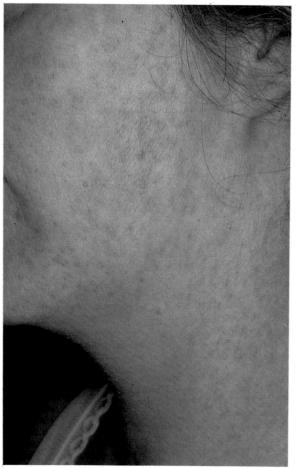

Figures 51 (left) and 52 (above)   Patient with serologically confirmed rubella with a rash on the neck and cheek and a red maculo-papular enanthem of the palate.

32

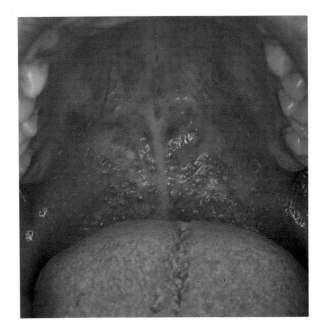

Figure 53 Koplik's spots on the palate.

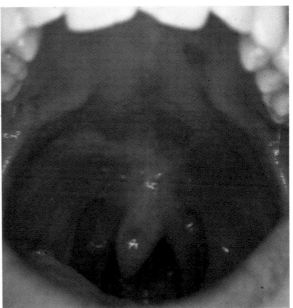

Figure 54 This blotchy uvulopalatal erythema in the mouth was eventually confirmed as infectious mononucleosis. Sore throats in teenagers should always be suspected as being glandular fever though the infectious mononucleosis tests are not always positive when first performed.

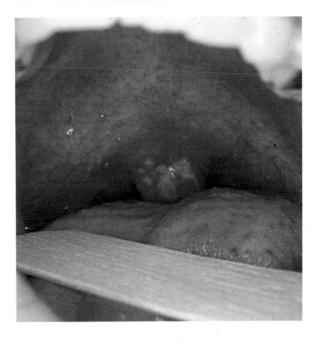

Figure 55 The uvula alone may be affected in glandular fever. No diagnosis was confirmed in this instance though evidence of infectious mononucleosis as well as herpes simplex and a streptococcus was sought.

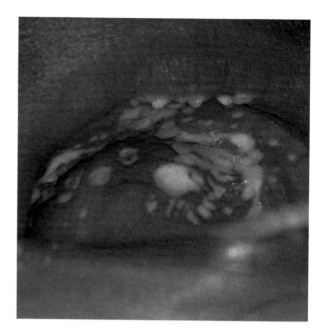

Figure 56 Thrush on the palate. Children with cystic fibrosis who often receive prolonged courses of antibiotics made up in sucrose syrups, are particularly prone to attacks.

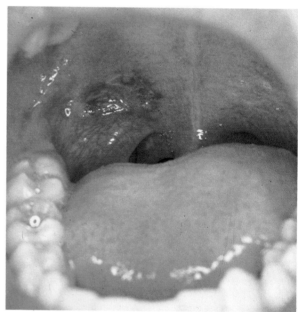

Figure 57 Injury sustained while sucking a pencil.

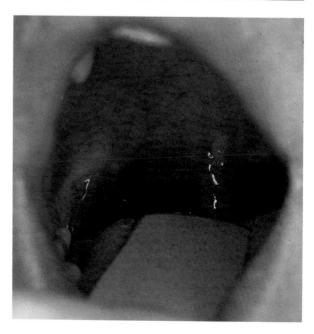

Figure 58 Injury caused by a sharp ball point pen piercing the palate.

5. THE TONSILS AND PHARYNX

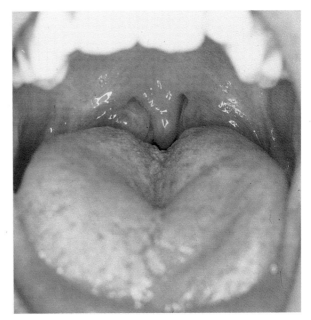

Figure 59 When examining the throat the physician will often only get a brief glimpse revealing no more than the uvula and upper part of the tonsils.

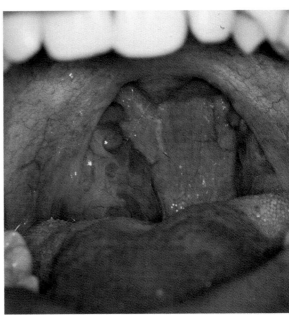

Figure 60 Very few children are able to control their tongue and soft palate to enable the tonsils and pharynx to be seen clearly as here. This shows a large right tonsil in an otherwise normal throat.

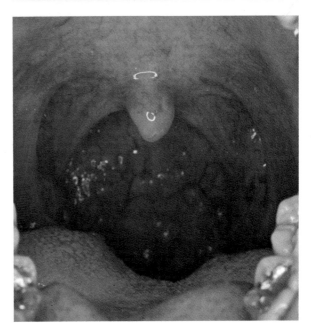

Figure 61 A common appearance of the lymphatic tissue on the posterior wall of the pharynx. This is normal and should not be confused with Steigman's lymphonodular pharyngitis.

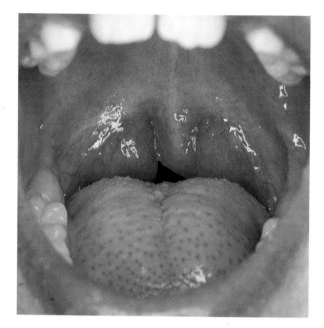

Figure 62 Large but normal tonsils preventing inspection of the pharynx.

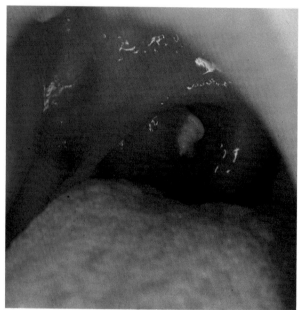

Figure 63 Cryptic debris of no pathological significance extruding from the right tonsil. The condition had been present for the previous six months and the child had remained well. The next figure provides a comparison.

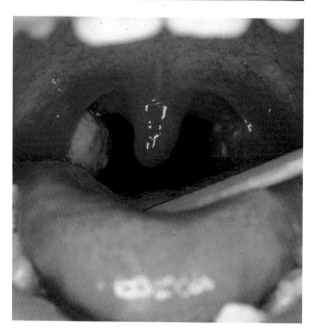

Figure 64 Exudative tonsillitis in infective mononucleosis.

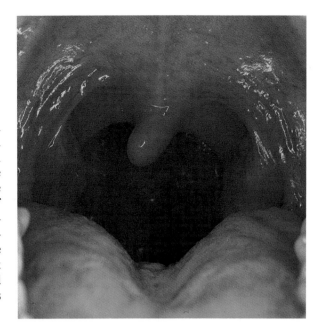

Figures 65 and 66 No tonsillar exudate can be seen here but the uvula, tonsils and pillars are a deep red and contrast with the normal colour of the buccal mucosa and palate. The clinician's problem with these cases is to decide whether streptococci are causing the inflammation. This appearance in the absence of other information has a 50% chance of being streptococcal. If there is submandibular tenderness (irrespective of whether lymph nodes can be felt or not) the chance rises to 65–70%. If in addition the patient has a frontal headache **and no cough**, the likelihood of a *β-haemolytic streptococcus* being the cause rises to 80%.

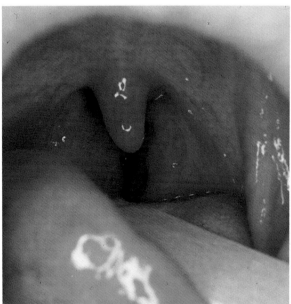

Figure 66

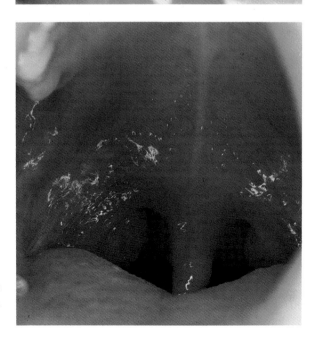

Figure 67 This streptococcal pharyngitis gives no extra hint of its bacterial cause. Note the papular rash on the soft palate.

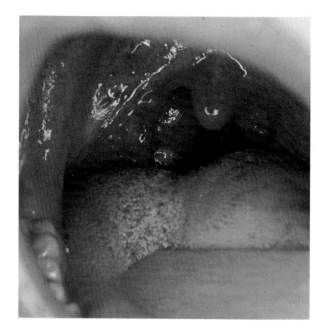

Figure 68 Acute streptococcal tonsillitis, again the throat appearance alone does not confirm a bacterial diagnosis. A throat culture or a probability check-list such as the one given with Figures 65 and 66 is the only way to reach a diagnosis.

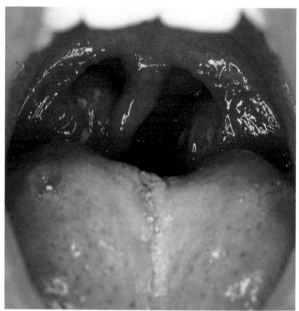

Figure 69 Exudative tonsillitis, in this case, streptococcal. The patient's age (16) suggested that it might be more likely due to infectious mononucleosis.

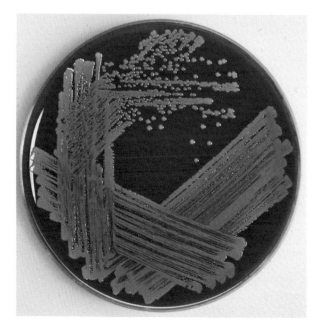

Figure 70 Culture of *Group A β-haemolytic streptococci.*

38

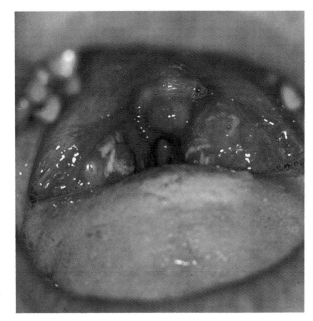

Figure 71 Exudative tonsillitis in infective mononucleosis.

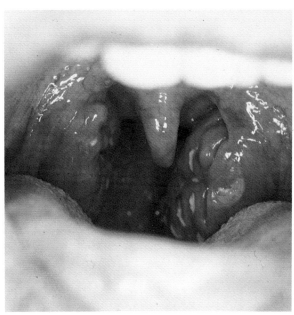

Figure 72 Frequent sore throats caused this patient to seek tonsillectomy. This illustrates her fourth attack in six months. The throat appearances were similar each time with exudate in the tonsillar crypts. Streptococci were isolated in the first and third attacks. This last attack, with an ulcer visible on the left tonsil, was due to infectious mononucleosis. The picture shows trismus: she could barely open her mouth.

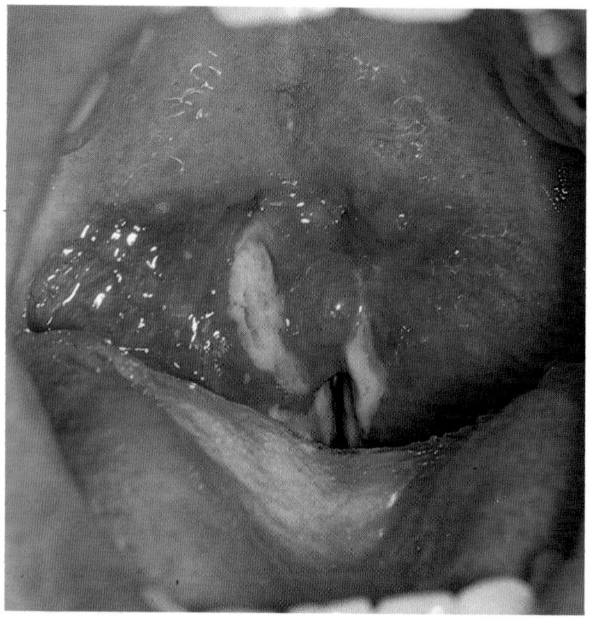

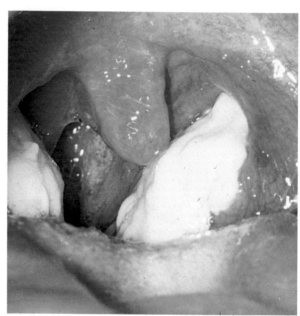

Figures 73 and 74 Exudative tonsillitis due to infectious mononucleosis. Halitosis is common with this condition but it occurs equally often in streptococcal disease. Tonsillar diphtheria is a possible explanation of gross exudate where the membrane is confined to the tonsils.

Figure 74

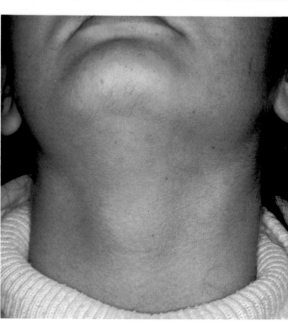

Figure 75 Enlarged submandibular lymph nodes due to infectious mononucleosis.

40

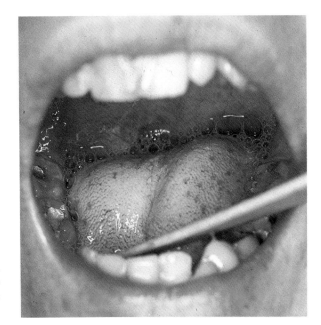

Figure 76 Unilateral tonsillar enlargement when accompanied by great tenderness and trismus is suggestive of quinsy, as in this case. It resolved with intramuscular penicillin without admission or tonsillectomy. A four year follow-up showed no recurrence.

The Question of Diagnosis

Apart from glandular fever, the only practical question for the primary care physician is "Is this throat inflammation due to streptococci?" Throat culture stands as the definitive answer, but it is a very specific test with a small proportion of false negatives and an even smaller proportion of false positives. Its drawbacks are obvious: delay and expense and at least three out of four negative cultures if all throats are swabbed. Because this book is an *Atlas*, the main stress has been on the visible physical signs, but the clinician must give weight to the presence or absence of neck tenderness just medial to the angle of the mandible, the presence or absence of headache and the group of respiratory (non-pharyngeal) symptoms of cough, running or blocked nose, and hoarseness, which are very helpful features in evaluating the likelihood of any one sore throat being streptococcal or non-streptococcal. The visible signs such as ulcers, petechiae and surface exudates suggest at once that we are not dealing with streptococci.

6. TONSILLECTOMY

Tonsillectomy is not a trivial operation and it should not be undertaken for tenuous reasons and without careful consideration of each individual case. The following sequence shows a tonsillectomy being performed on a 5-year-old. The surgeon's view is from above and behind with the patient's neck fully extended.

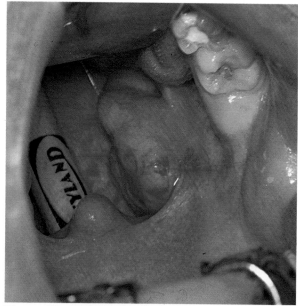

Figure 77   Endotracheal tube prior to incision.

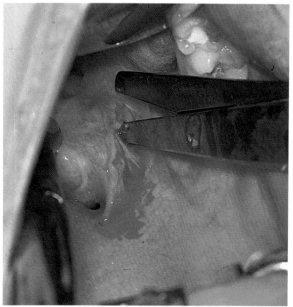

Figure 78   An incision is made with scissors.

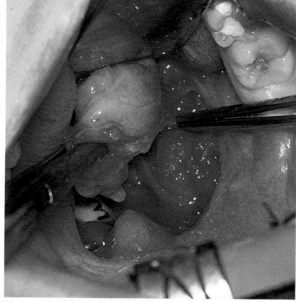

Figure 79   Tonsil dissection.

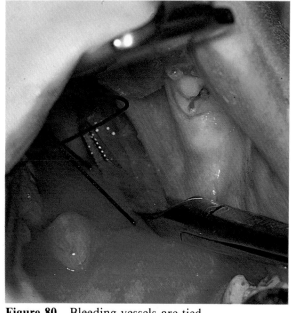

Figure 80   Bleeding vessels are tied.

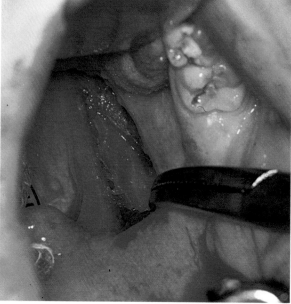

Figure 81   Tonsillar bed at completion of operation.

PART 2. EAR DISORDERS

1. ANATOMY

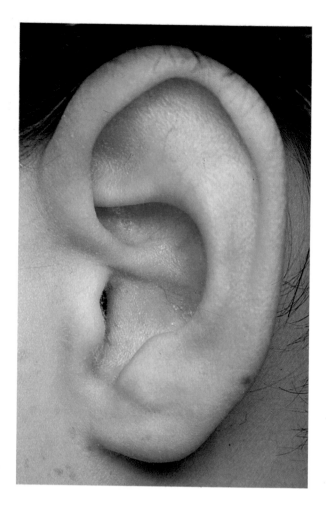

Figure 82 The auricle, also known as the pinna, is a skin covered elastic fibro-cartilaginous plate.

Figures 83 (opposite, top) and 84 (opposite, bottom) The external auditory canal is a slightly curved structure with its concavity facing downwards and forwards. It is composed of two portions – an external part which is cartilaginous and an inner part which is formed by bone. The tympanic membrane is set obliquely at the inner end of the external auditory canal in such a way that the roof and exterior wall are shorter than the floor and anterior wall. It is convex towards the tympanic cavity. It consists of three layers – an outer epithelial layer, a middle fibrous layer, and an inner mucosal layer. The eustachian tube is more horizontal and relatively wider and shorter in the child than in the adult. The upper third of the eustachian tube is bony, with the lower two thirds cartilaginous. The opening into the lateral wall of the nasopharynx lies on a level with the inferior turbinate.

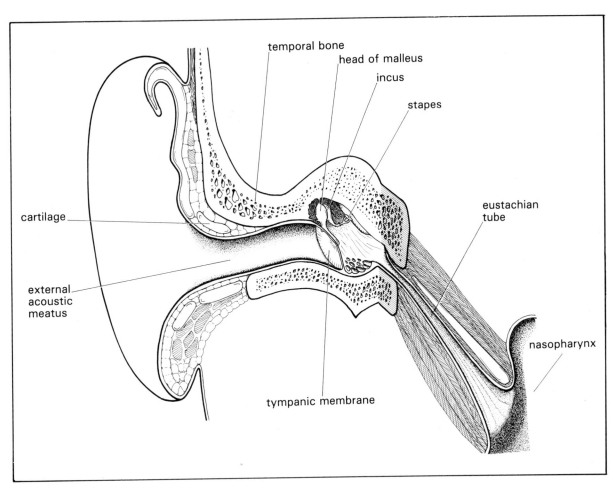

temporal bone
head of malleus
incus
stapes
eustachian tube
nasopharynx
tympanic membrane
cartilage
external acoustic meatus

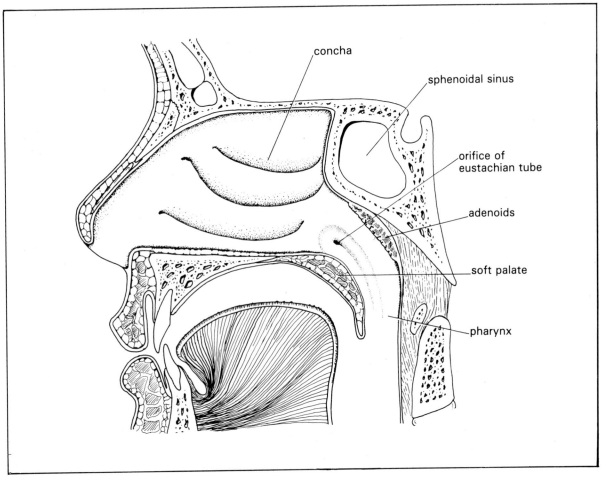

concha
sphenoidal sinus
orifice of eustachian tube
adenoids
soft palate
pharynx

Figure 85 The normal tympanic membrane is thin and semi-transparent. When viewed through an otoscope it has a pearly-grey appearance and often some structures within the middle ear, such as the long process of the incus and the opening of the eustachian tube, can be seen if it is sufficiently transparent. Where the outer margin of the drum is attached to the external canal it is thickened and called the annulus fibrosa. The upper one-fifth of the drum is slack and called the pars flaccida and the lower four-fifths called the pars tensa. The handle of the malleus, which extends downwards and backwards, is a reliable landmark. The short process of the malleus protrudes forwards into the external canal. The umbo is the central attachment of the tympanic membrane to the malleus. From the umbo a cone of light extends downwards and forwards. The blood supply of the tympanic membrane comes from the ear canal superiorly. Prominent blood vessels on the rim superiorly are within normal limits.

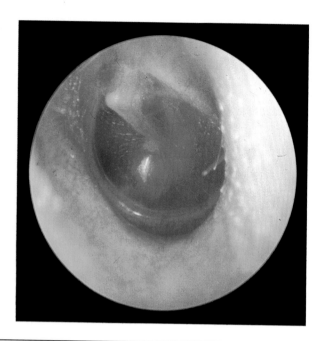

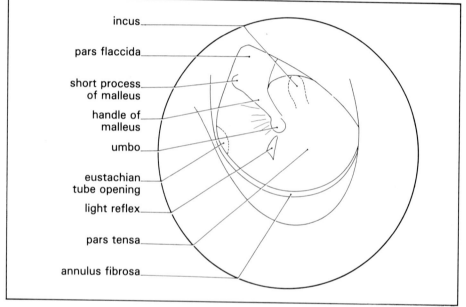

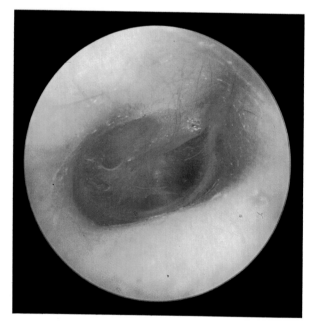

Figure 86 A leash of blood vessels often extends over the malleus and this sign should not lead to the assumption that infection is present. Examination of the ear with an otoscope can result in reflex dilatation of blood vessels in the eardrum and syringing of the ear can also cause a temporary increase in vascularity of the drum.

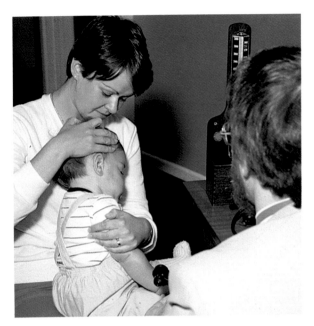

Figure 87 When examining younger children, it is advisable to have the child sitting on the parent's knee with the mother gently restricting the child's arm with one hand and with firm application of the other to the child's head.

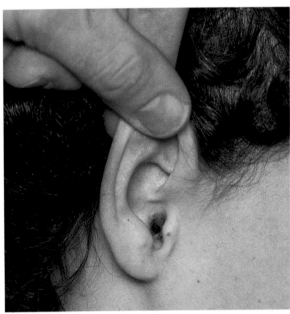

Figure 88 On examining a child's ear, the auricle should be drawn gently upwards and backwards. This should straighten the meatus and help to reveal the tympanic membrane.

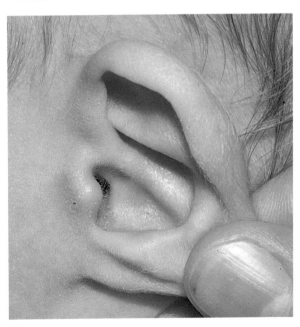

Figure 89 In young infants it is often necessary to pull the auricle downwards and backwards during examination.

2. LOOKING INTO THE EAR

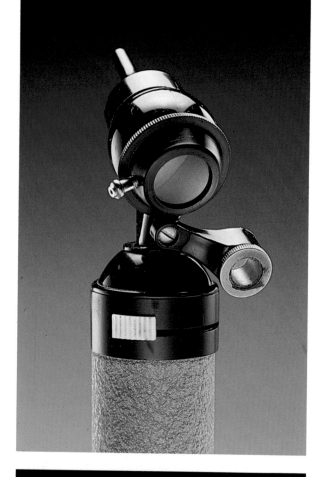

Figure 90 The electric otoscope (or auriscope) is the instrument most commonly used by primary care physicians. It is important to ensure that the batteries function and the speculae are kept clean. A speculum should be selected that is the largest that can be inserted without causing pain.

Figure 91 Assessment of drum mobility is best done in the consulting room with the pneumatic otoscope. This is a standard otoscope with attached tube and bulb. By observing the tympanic membrane as the bulb is alternately squeezed and released in rapid succession the degree of eardrum mobility and response to both positive and negative pressure can be estimated. This estimation can often be critical in an assessment of middle ear function.

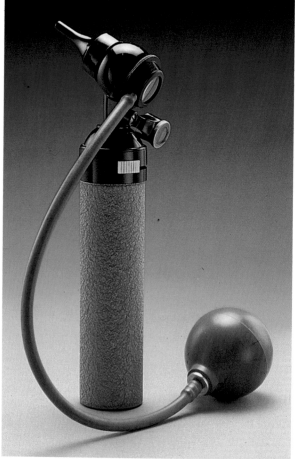

Adam Rouilly (London) Ltd, in conjunction with the authors, have produced a model head for practising ear examination techniques. The model comprises a mounted head with a flexible ear incorporating an accurately modelled outer meatus. It contains reproductions of pictures used in this book which are positioned in a realistic manner within the head for viewing with an auriscope. Full details from: Adam Rouilly (London) Ltd, Crown Quay Lane, Sittingbourne, Kent ME10 3JG.

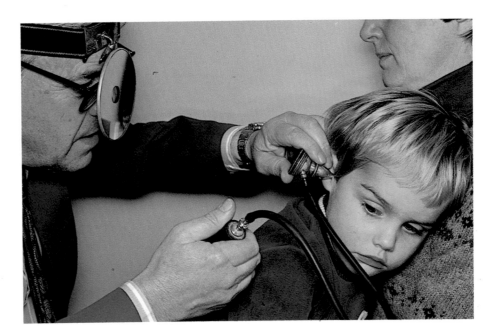

Figure 92 Where pneumatic otoscopy is considered an important part of routine examination, Seigle's apparatus is a valuable addition to the instruments to be used in examination of the ear. This apparatus allows magnification through an obliquely set lens and mobility of the drum head can be determined by alternate compression and release of the bulb.

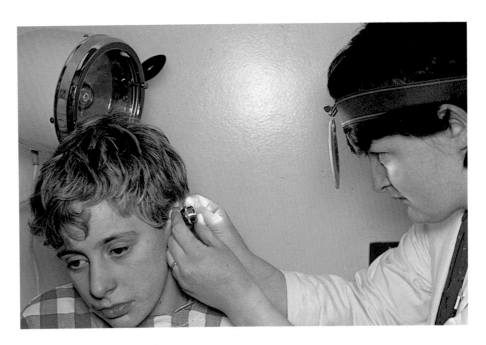

Figure 93 The examination of the ear with the help of a head mirror is done with the child and the examiner in a sitting position. The light source should be behind and to the side of the patient's head which should be turned to one side and tilted away from the examiner so that the ear is readily accessible.

3. HEARING TESTS

There are three organic types of deafness – conductive, sensorineural and mixed. Conductive deafness is due to any lesion of the conductivity apparatus and can be caused by obstruction or defect of the external meatus, tympanic membrane, middle ear cavity or ossicles. Sensorineural deafness is caused by lesions affecting the receiving apparatus and defects of the cochlea or auditory nerve. In mixed deafness, conductive and sensorineural causes are both present in the same ear.

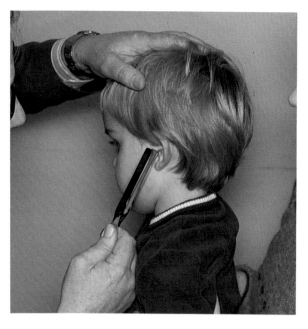

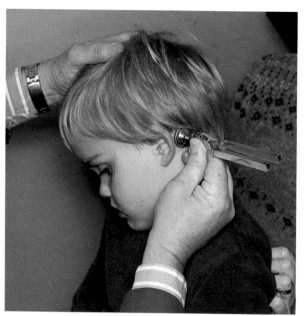

Figures 94 (above), 95 (above right) and 96 (right)
Rinne's test is performed with a 512 Hz tuning fork which is gently struck on a soft surface and then held close to the external auditory meatus. When the child indicates that it can no longer be heard, the base of the tuning fork is placed on the mastoid process and if the patient cannot hear it, it is a positive or normal Rinne's test, indicating that air conduction is better than bone conduction. In assessing bone conduction, it is important to avoid touching the posterior wall of the canal. If the patient can hear the tuning fork when it is placed on the mastoid process, after he can no longer hear it by air conduction this is a negative Rinne's test, indicating bone conduction is better than air conduction and hence the child is suffering from conductive deafness.

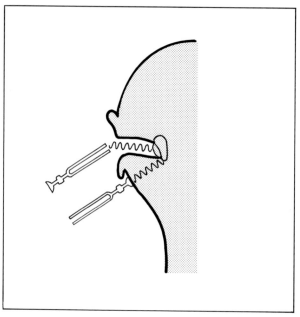

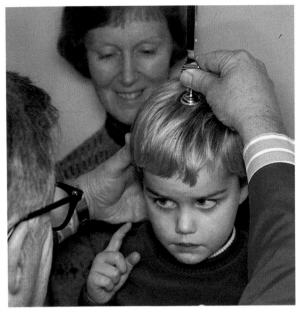

Figures 97 and 98 An alternative, although less reliable, test is Weber's test where the base of the fork is held on the vertex in the mid line and the patient is asked in which ear he is hearing the sound. In conductive deafness sound is referred to the deaf ear, and in sensorineural deafness the sound is referred to the non-affected ear. If the patient's hearing is normal or equally diminished in both ears there will be no lateralisation of sound.

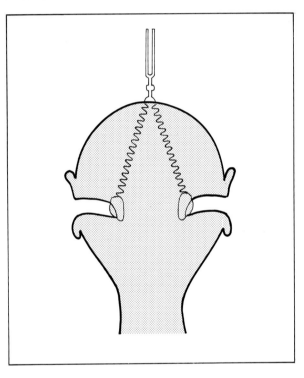

Figure 98

Figures 99, 100 and 101 Active cooperation in hearing tests is not always easy in children. Younger children are normally seated on their mother's knee and their attention held by one examiner who also observes any responses. A second person makes a variety of noises out of sight of the child and by using sounds of different pitches and loudness an assessment of hearing can be made. Suitable sounds are produced by the crinkling of crisp thin paper, shaking a rattle, or by stroking a spoon gently round the inside of a cup.

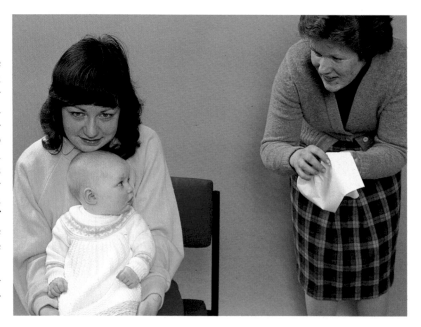

Figure 100

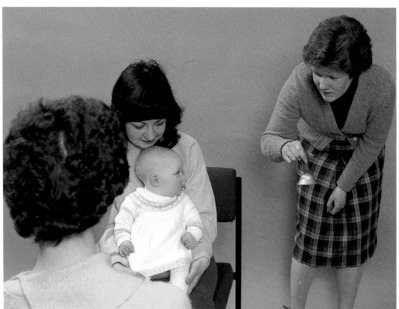

Figure 101

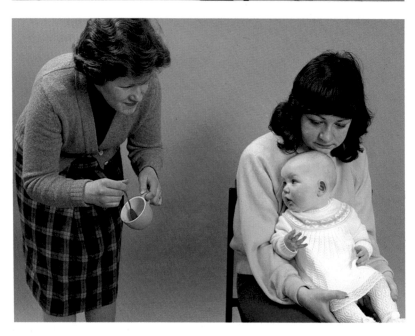

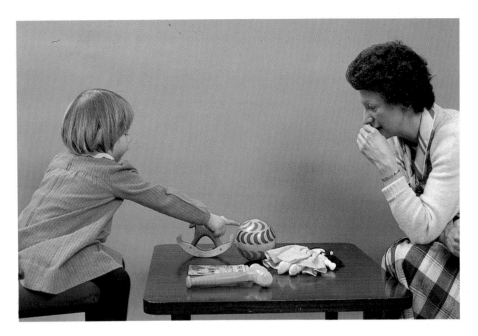

Figure 102 In the older child, the clinical methods most commonly employed in assessment are the ticking watch, the forced whisper and conversational voice test. The whispered voice test is preferred to the ticking watch because it covers the spectrum of frequencies used in normal speech. It can be a good screening test and can identify hearing deficits of 15 to 20 decibels or more. One way to carry out the test is to arrange a number of recognisable toys in front of the child. The examiner then faces the child with her mouth covered, and using a whisper asks the child to point to or pick up individual toys.

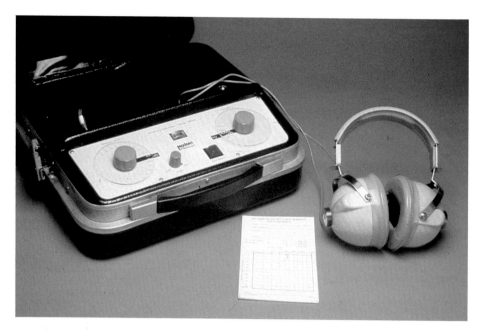

Figure 103 Audiometry can be carried out in the majority of children aged 4 or over. The audiometer is an electronic instrument which delivers pure tone stimuli to the ear at frequencies from 125 Hz to 8000 Hz. For full audiological assessment it is necessary to deliver test tones through earphones to either ear.

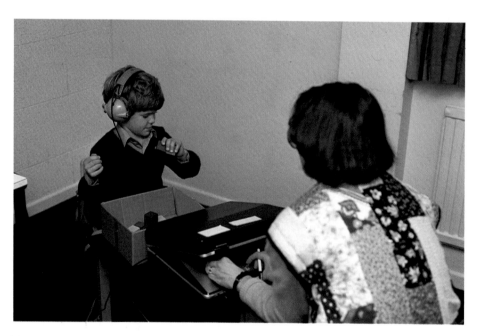

Figure 104 Testing should be conducted in a quiet room, preferably treated for sound exclusion. The child is told to place a brick in the box when he hears the tone. It is important that the audiometer is calibrated at least annually.

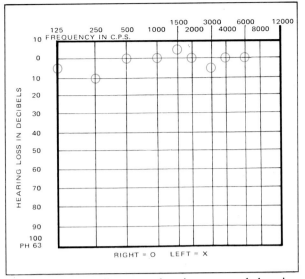

Figure 105 Audiogram showing normal hearing right ear.

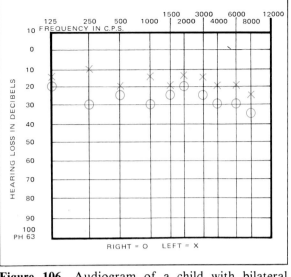

Figure 106 Audiogram of a child with bilateral moderate hearing loss.

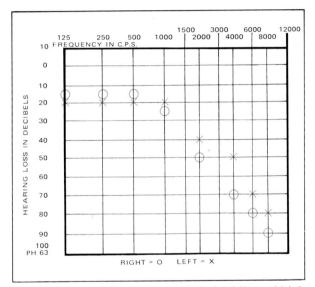

Figure 107 Audiogram of a child with bilateral high tone deafness.

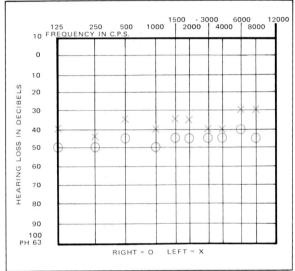

Figure 108 Audiogram of a child with conductive deafness due to secretory otitis media.

Figure 109 Electric acoustic impedance testing and, in particular, tympanometry, are more sensitive methods for detecting middle ear effusion in children. The apparatus used is shown here. In tympanometry, the external canal is converted into a closed chamber and a fixed frequency tone is delivered into the canal. The ear pressure is then varied and this alters the stiffness of the tympanic membrane and the reflection of sound from its surface.

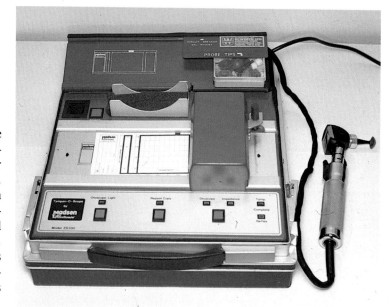

Figure 110 Measurements of eardrum impedance are recorded as a graphic display or tympanogram which provides objective measurements of eardrum mobility. The result expected from a normal ear is illustrated here. (A) indicates the peak middle ear pressure and (B) indicates the compliance of 0.7 ml which is within normal range. (C) is an indicator mark for the compliance scale used to note the compliance of the middle ear system. (D) represents the measured volume in ml of the ear canal. The presence of an ipsilateral reflex is shown in the section on the right.

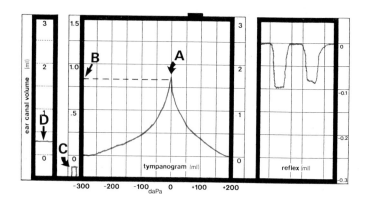

Figure 111 This tympanogram was obtained from a child with serous otitis media. Note the flat shape of the curve, normal ear canal volume and lack of a peak pressure point. The acoustic reflex is absent in such cases.

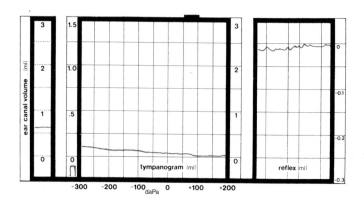

4. THE EXTERNAL AUDITORY MEATUS

i. Wax

Figures 112, 113, 114 and 115 Wax, or cerumen, is a normal secretion in the cerumenous glands in the outer part of the meatus, and can obscure or partially obscure the drum. When it is first produced it is colourless and semi-liquid in consistency, but with time it changes from pale yellow, to golden yellow, to light brown and finally, black. As the wax darkens it also hardens, and the darker the colour the denser the consistency.

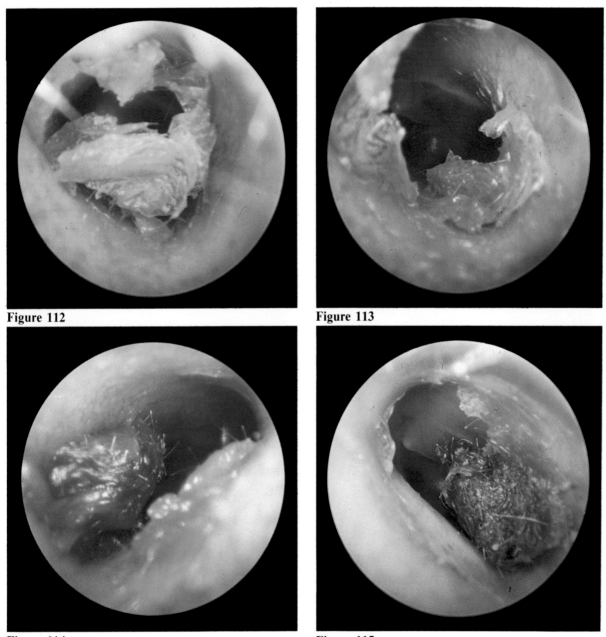

Figure 112

Figure 113

Figure 114

Figure 115

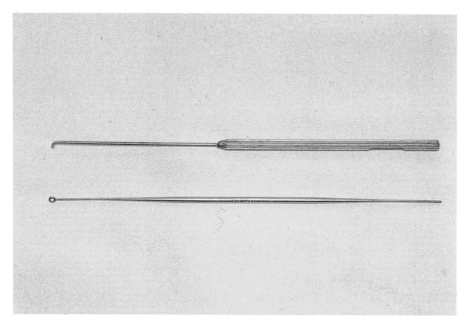

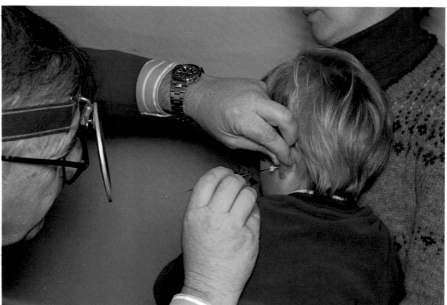

Figures 116 and 117 If produced in large quantities, wax may form an impacted mass causing deafness and sometimes irritation of the meatal lining. It can often be removed quite easily by using a wax hook or a probe with cotton wool attached.

Figure 118 Syringing. The metal syringe is the traditional model and several nozzles should be available to allow continued use of the syringe while contaminated nozzles are being sterilised. If the plunger is occasionally removed and lubricated with soft soap or silicone solution, performance is improved. Removal of wax can be facilitated by the use of sodium bicarbonate ear drops for one week prior to gentle syringing. This will avoid the possibility of causing distress to a young child who may be upset by vigorous syringing.

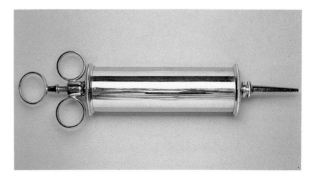

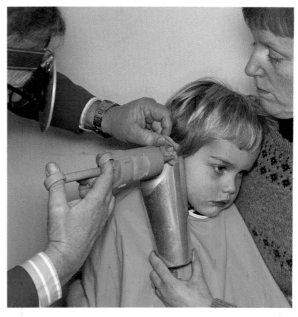

Figure 119 An improved syringe has recently been marketed constructed from polypropylene, which is rigid up to 130°C. The plunger is provided with two neoprene rings which give a smooth leakproof action. Syringing should be carried out with water at 37°C. Any variation in water temperature of more than a few degrees may cause vertigo. Towels are used to protect the patient's clothing. The pinna is pulled upwards and backwards to straighten the ear canal.

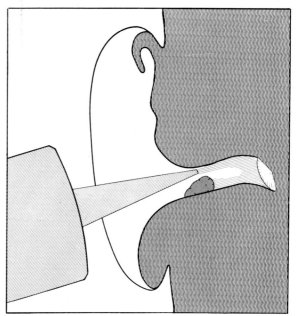

Figure 120 The nozzle of the syringe is pointed upwards and slightly posteriorly to project the stream beyond the wax. Moderate pressure should be applied to the plunger and every effort made to maintain a constant flow of water.

ii. Foreign Bodies

All sorts of foreign bodies are introduced into the external auditory meatus by small children; the chief danger lies in clumsy attempts at removal. If the child is uncooperative a general anaesthetic may be required. Some small foreign bodies can often be removed by syringing but removal of vegetable matter by syringing is contraindicated because of the danger of the material absorbing water and swelling.

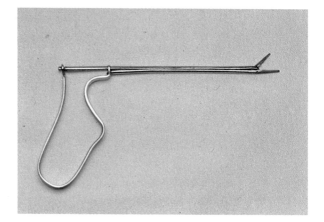

Figures 121 and 122 If the object is superficial it may be possible to grasp it with crocodile forceps or extract it with a wax hook. Using a head mirror for illumination, the foreign body can be gently grasped and extracted easily.

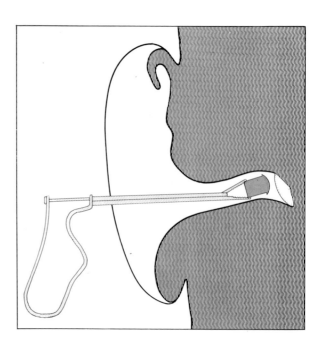

Figure 122

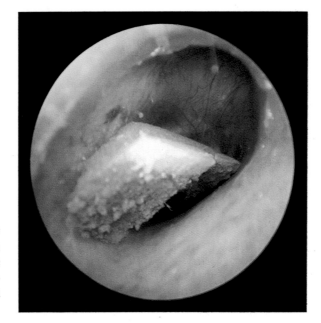

Figure 123 Small objects can often be removed by syringing but larger foreign bodies such as this section of an eraser which virtually fills the lumen may be pushed further in by syringing or attempts at extraction. Removal involved hospital admission for a general anaesthetic.

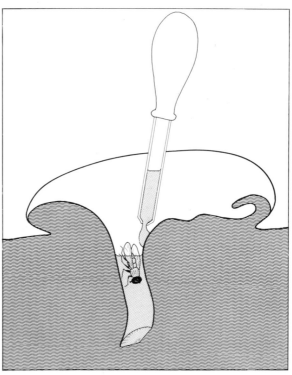

Figure 124 Insects should be first killed by using a few drops of oil or spirit and thereafter removed by syringing.

iii. Otitis Externa and Eczema

Otitis externa is an acute or chronic reaction of the skin of the external canal to a variety of agents which may be bacterial, fungal, viral or chemical. Otitis externa may also be due to eczema or seborrhoeic dermatitis.

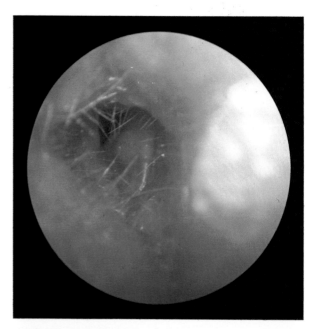

Figure 125 Otitis externa causing almost total obstruction of the ear canal.

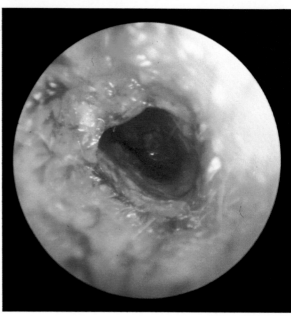

Figure 126 Moist debris in the canal with underlying oedema of the meatal skin.

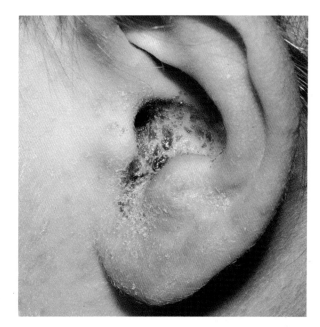

Figure 127 Seborrhoeic dermatitis and inflammation of the pinna. Same child as Figure 126.

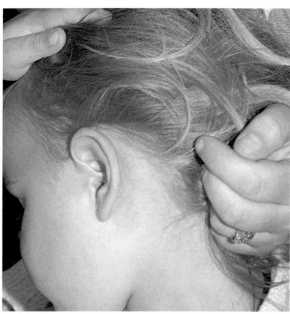

Figure 128 Seborrhoeic dermatitis which has extended behind the pinna.

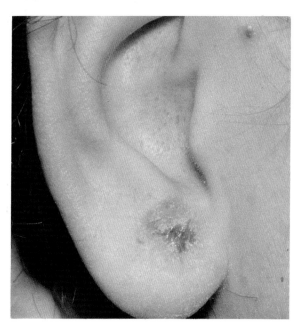

Figure 129 Skin reaction after attempted ear piercing.

5. THE TYMPANIC MEMBRANE AND MIDDLE EAR CAVITY

i. Acute Otitis Media

Acute otitis media is almost invariably the result of inflammation of the middle ear cavity accompanied by obstruction of the eustachian tube. Where bacteria can be recovered from the middle ear fluid, *Streptococcus pneumoniae* and *Haemophilus influenzae* are two of the most frequently isolated organisms. Of the the two, *Streptococcus pneumoniae* is found more commonly irrespective of age. Although *Haemophilus influenzae* is more likely to occur in younger rather than older children it is consistently less likely to be the cause of infection than *Streptococcus pneumoniae*. Other organisms and viruses are much less frequently isolated and in about twenty-five per cent of middle ear infection no organisms are cultured.

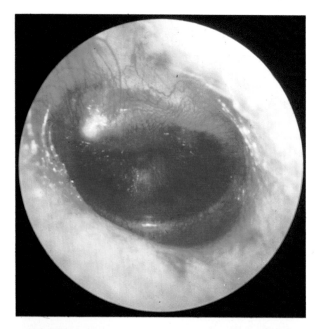

Figure 130 Acute otitis media in a 3-year-old. The tympanic membrane has lost its lustre and blood vessels are prominent along the periphery. As the condition progressed the drum became profusely red.

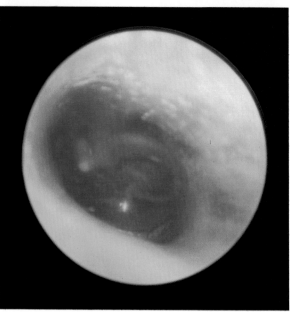

Figure 131 Inflammation of the drum accompanied by middle ear effusion which shows as fluid levels on the tympanic membrane.

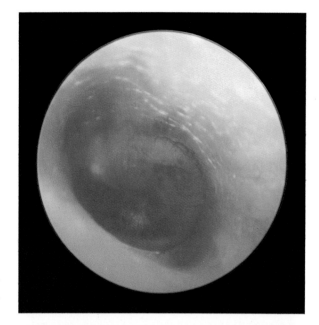

Figure 132 Erythema with prominent vessels obvious round the handle of the malleus. This condition persisted for two weeks.

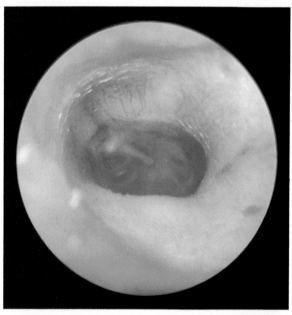

Figure 133 In some instances after acute otitis media, middle ear effusion may persist for several weeks. In this case effusion, indicated by fluid levels below the malleus, lasted for six weeks.

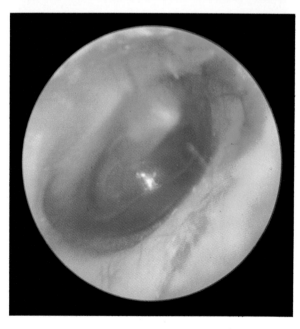

Figure 134 A 4-year-old after the onset of earache. The tympanic membrane is erythematous with slight bulging of the drum and a fluid line indicating effusion.

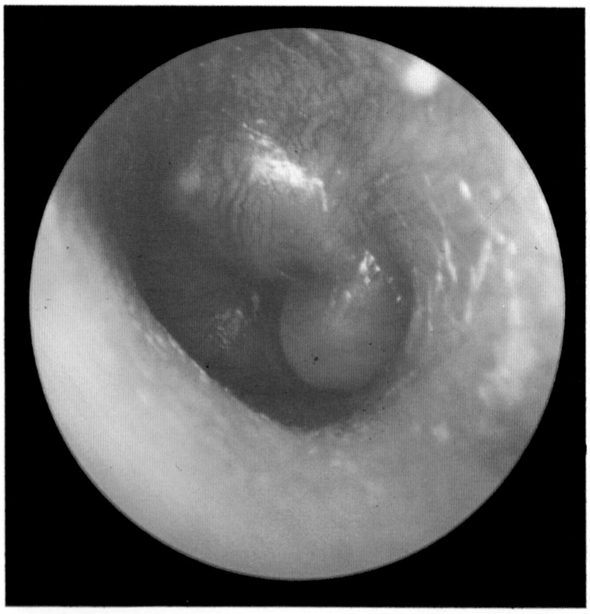

Figures 135 and 136 Acute purulent otitis media accompanied by considerable bulging of the drum with purulent material behind the tense tympanic membrane and this appearance occasionally heralds perforation. Ten days later the majority of abnormalities have cleared, but there is still evidence of middle ear effusion (Figure 136).

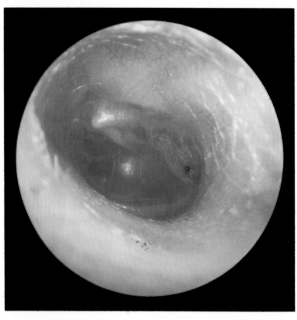

Figure 136

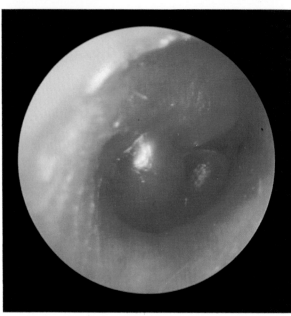

Figure 137 An acutely inflamed bulging drum with no recognisable landmarks.

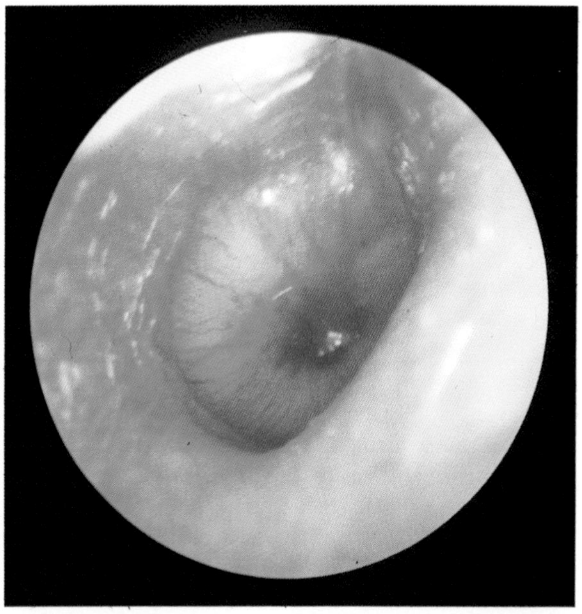

Figures 138 and 139 A 7-year-old with otitis media with erythema and bulging of the drum on the periphery. Two weeks later the inflammation had resolved, no fluid was present, and the tympanic membrane had returned to normal (Figure 139).

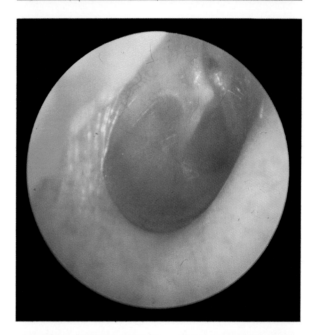

Figure 139

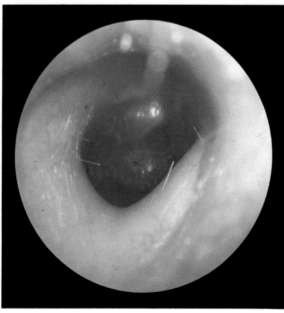

Figure 140 In this ear a number of bullae can be seen on the surface of the drum and appearances are described as bullous myringitis. This is probably not a specific clinical entity, but merely acute otitis media with blisters on the drum, evidence of association with mycoplasma pneumoniae or specific viruses being weak or doubtful.

ii. Serous Otitis Media

Serous otitis media (glue ear) is often seen as a sequel to recurrent acute otitis media. It may also occur without a previous history of acute infection. The affected ear may be deaf but the level of deafness is not constant. Nevertheless careful assessment of hearing is essential. Those who are not deaf need follow-up but not necessarily treatment. Eustachian tube obstruction results in failure to replace the air which is normally absorbed by the wall of the middle ear. This results in lowering of the middle ear pressure with consequent effusion of fluid. Serous otitis media is often the result of eustachian insufficiency but not all cases of middle ear effusion are due to eustachian tube blockage; viral and allergic causes can also contribute.

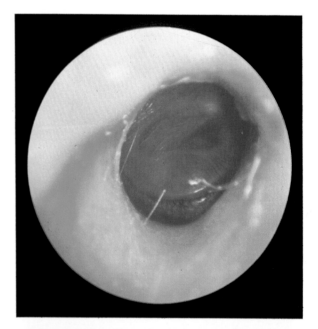

Figure 141 An effusion is visible through the eardrum with a fluid meniscus defining the upper margin.

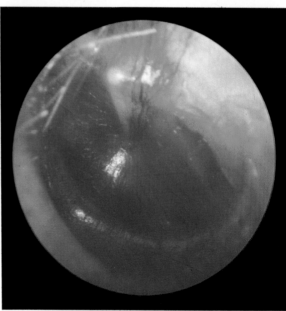

Figure 142 The appearance of secretory otitis media prior to incision for myringotomy.

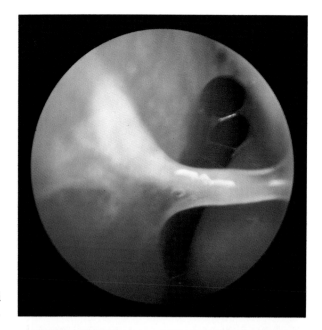

Figure 143 Thick mucus seen in the **nose** of a child with serous otitis media; a frequently associated sign.

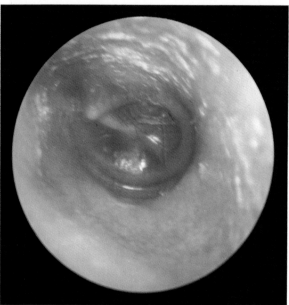

Figure 144 Eustachian tube obstruction results in failure of replacement of air which is normally absorbed from the middle ear, and this results in vacuum formation, and, as shown here, in-drawing of the drum and effusion of fluid.

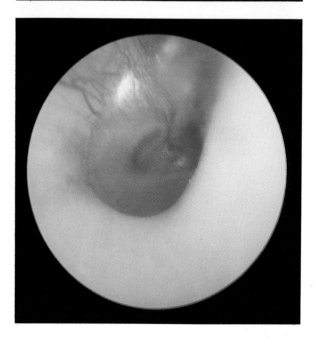

Figure 145 Early serous otitis media showing a slight yellow tinge to the drum with the annular and radial blood vessels injected. In cases of chronic effusion, amber-coloured fluid can be visualised behind the drum.

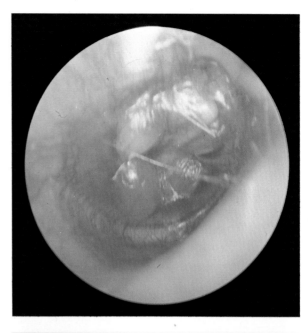

Figures 146, 147 and 148 In this series, the appearance of the tympanic membrane is shown in a 7-year-old child who presented with pain and deafness in the right ear. The tympanic membrane was distorted by middle ear effusion and glue (Figure 146). Two days later, there was some improvement with the handle of the malleus visible, although characteristically foreshortened and horizontal (Figure 147). One week later the main finding was a retracted drum (Figure 148).

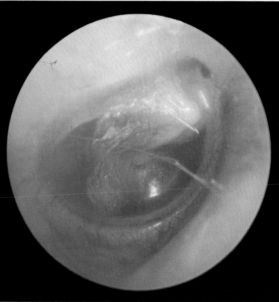

Figure 147

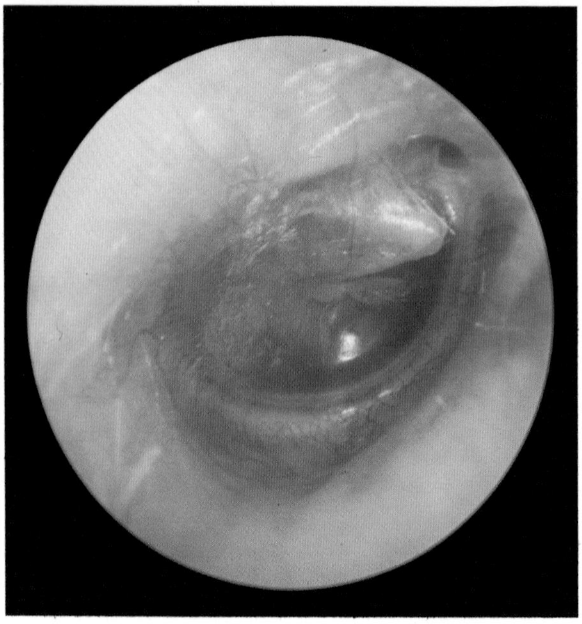

Figure 148

70

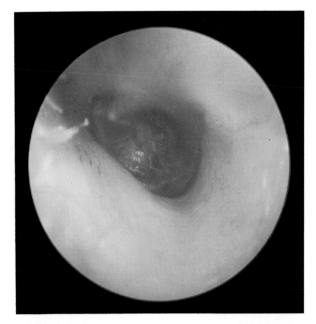

Figure 149 A further example of a retracted drum.

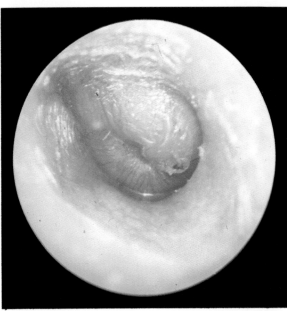

Figure 150 A longstanding case of middle ear effusion. There are considerable changes in the appearance of the drum with the normal landmarks not visible and glue-like secretions distorting the drum.

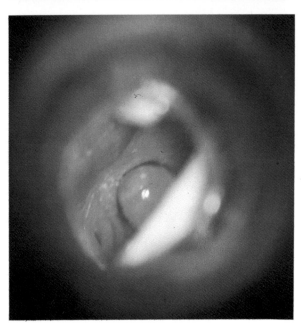

Figure 151 Macroscopically, 'glue' has the appearance of mucus and is pale grey or yellow. This is the appearance seen through a speculum following a myringotomy.

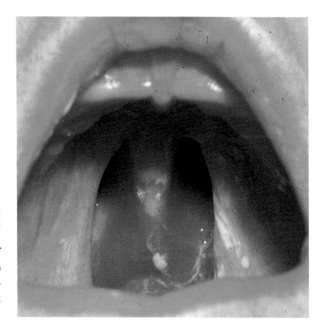

Figure 152 Cleft palate in an infant prior to repair. Glue ear is common in children with cleft palate, even after the defect has been repaired. Otitis media is virtually universal among infants with cleft palate. Possible explanations include (a) abnormality of structure and function of the eustachian tube, (b) disturbance of aerodynamic and hydrodynamic relationships in the nasopharynx and the proximal part of the eustachian tube.

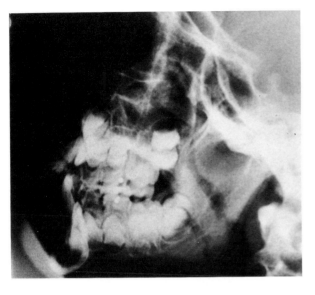 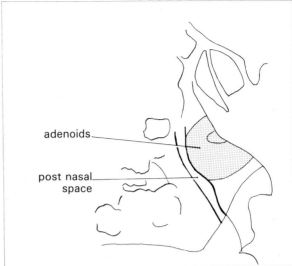

Figure 153 **Hypertrophy of the adenoids** is a common cause of tubal obstruction in children either by obstruction of the tubal openings or by reducing post-nasal space. This 6-year-old boy had considerable nasal obstruction, a history of frequent upper respiratory tract infection and recurrent otitis media. The X-ray shows that the adenoids are generally enlarged causing significant narrowing of the post-nasal space. Following adenoidectomy considerable improvement occurred and he had no otitis media in the two years after operation.

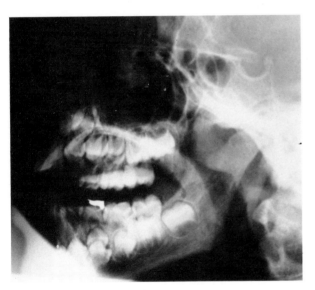 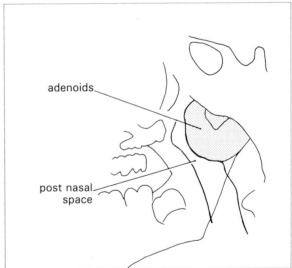

Figure 154 This 8-year-old boy had a history of frequent otitis media since the age of 3, accompanied by partial hearing loss. The X-ray shows prominent adenoids with localised obstruction of the post-nasal airway.

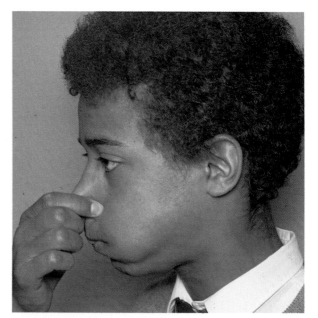

Figure 155 Valsalva's manoeuvre. Resolution of effusion will occur by drainage down the eustachian canal. One measure which is often found useful is inflation of the middle ear by Valsalva's manoeuvre. This can be performed by older children who pinch the nostrils between forefinger and thumb then, with lips tightly compressed, blow the cheeks out.

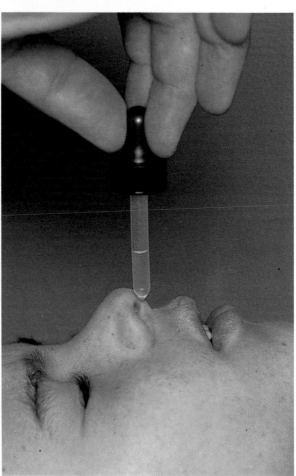

Figure 156 Decongestant nose drops may succeed in some cases. They should not be used for more than two weeks because they eventually provoke irreversible change to the mucous membrane of the nose.

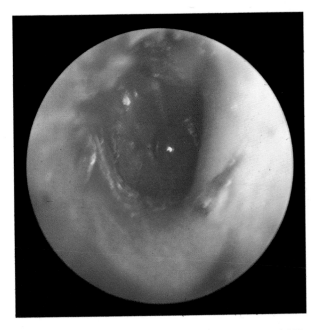

Figure 157 **Myringotomy** can be used to treat middle ear effusion where a small incision is made behind and below the handle of the malleus. The picture shows a bleb of purulent effusion welling up through the incision. In many cases myringotomy combined with Valsalva's manoeuvre will result in evacuation of the middle ear effusion.

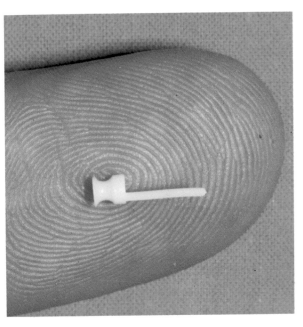

Figure 158 **Grommets** can be inserted in the tympanic membrane if medical treatment and myringotomy are unsuccessful and the child has persistent middle ear effusion. Grommets, or tympanostomy tubes, are silicone tubes retained in an opening in the drum by inner and outer flanges.

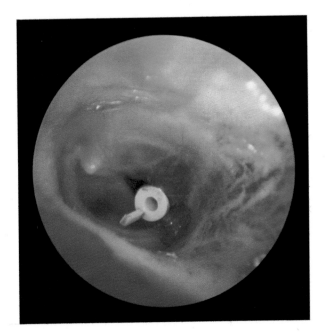

Figure 159 A grommet in place. The most important function of the grommet is to equalise the air pressure on both sides of the tympanic membrane. This creates an artificial eustachian tube to ventilate the middle ear.

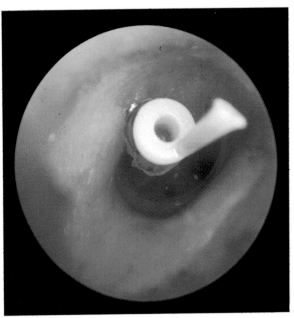

Figure 160 An extruded grommet adhering to the side of the external canal. Grommets are spontaneously extruded at about 6–12 months after insertion.

iii. Early Tympanosclerosis

In some cases of otitis media healing may not be complete and the inflammatory process leads to formation of scar tissue. This can take the form of calcified plaques on the tympanic membrane.

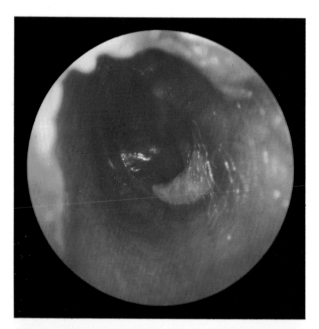

Figure 161 A mild case of tympanosclerosis. Small patches are present in the tympanic membrane and hearing is not affected.

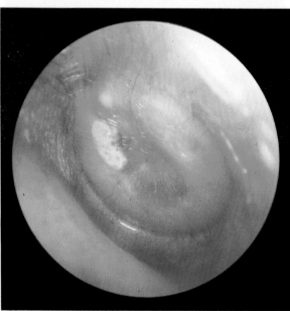

Figure 162 A more severe case of early tympanosclerosis. Most of the drum is affected, there is impaired mobility and conductive hearing loss.

iv. Perforations

Perforations are usually single but may be multiple. Spontaneous rupture of the tympanic membrane can occur in association with acute infection when the tense eardrum perforates and releases pus. In some children recurrent infection with associated perforations may result in persistent and ultimately permanent perforation. There are three main types of perforation and they are referred to as central, marginal and attic. Perforations of the pars flaccida are called attic and perforations of the pars tensa are called central.

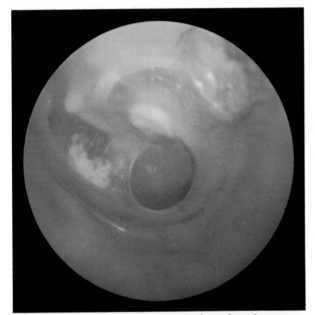

Figure 163 Longstanding central perforation.

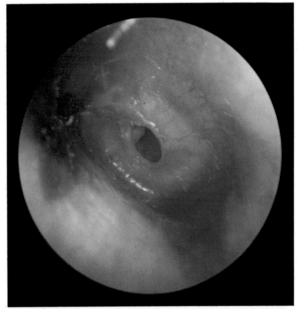

Figure 164 Central perforation.

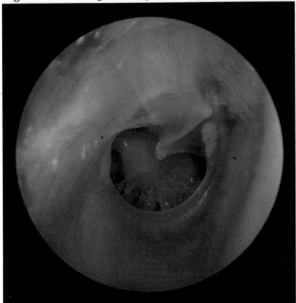

Figure 165 Very large central perforations such as this are described as sub-total.

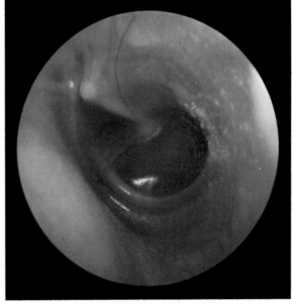

Figure 166 Patch of transparent drum. This appearance can be mistaken for a perforation.

6. ILLUSTRATED CASE HISTORIES OF FIVE CHILDREN WITH EAR PROBLEMS

Case One

Angela had her first episode of bilateral otitis media at the age of 30 months, and during the next 18 months had recurrent attacks of infection culminating in insertion of grommets at the age of four. Following removal of the grommets she had no problems for 6 months until the age of 5 when she had an episode of right otitis media with congestion of the drum and there was difficulty in visualising the handle of the malleus (Figure 167). Four days later (Figure 168) there was a slight improvement in appearance with the handle of the malleus more readily visible. At this stage she had partial deafness in the right ear.

During the next two months she remained well but, although asymptomatic, the appearance of the tympanic membrane (Figure 169) was suggestive of middle ear effusion with the handle of the malleus more horizontal than normal. Follow-up examination two months later revealed a tympanic membrane which had a much improved appearance (Figure 170). She had been without problems for over two months, and her hearing was normal.

Three months later, at the age of 6 years, she had a flare-up of symptoms with right earache, fever, cough and a congested drum (Figure 171) all of which responded rapidly to antibiotics. She progressed satisfactorily and follow-up examination two months later revealed that hearing was normal, but the right tympanic membrane (Figure 172) was still suggestive of middle ear effusion.

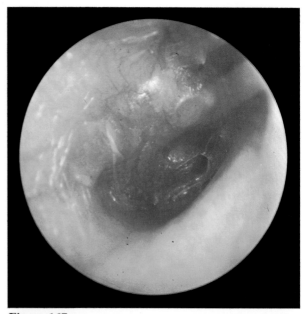

Figure 167

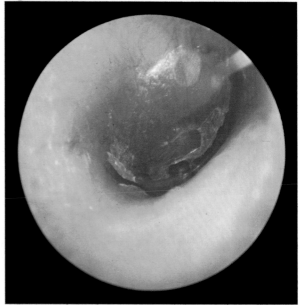

Figure 168

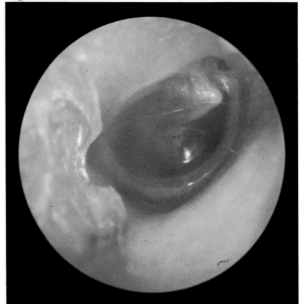

Figure 169

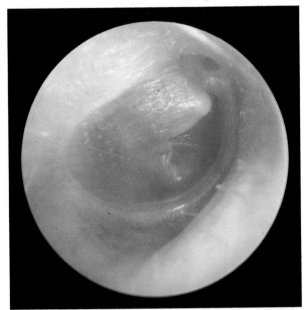

Figure 170

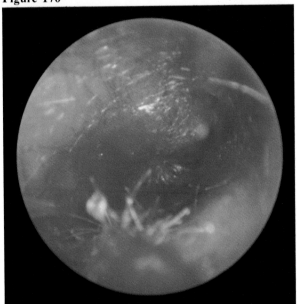

Figure 171

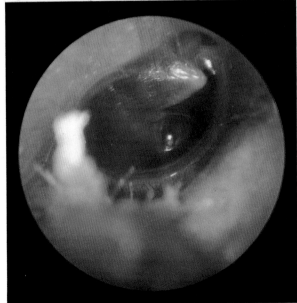

Figure 172

Case Two

Otitis media is common in families. Alan, Angela's brother (see Case 1) had his first episode of left acute otitis media aged 1 year and in the ensuing three years, he had 13 episodes of middle ear infection requiring medical care. The infections responded rapidly to treatment with antibiotics and he had no hearing problems. Figure 173 shows his left eardrum three weeks after an acute infection when he was aged 3. The drum was dull and he had partial hearing loss in the left ear.

In the next six months, he had only one episode of respiratory tract infection and eardrum appearances were much improved (Figure 174).

At the age of 5 years he had a further episode of bilateral earache (Figures 175 and 176), but this quickly resolved with both ears within normal limits.

Despite a history of recurrent upper respiratory tract infection and otitis media, Alan's hearing was not affected and his eardrums quickly returned to normal following the attacks.

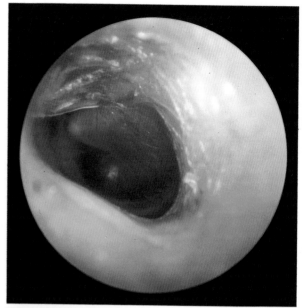

Figure 173

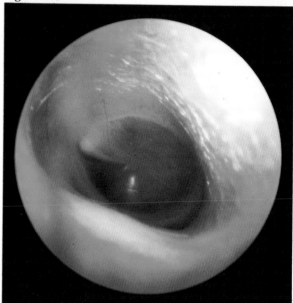

Figure 174

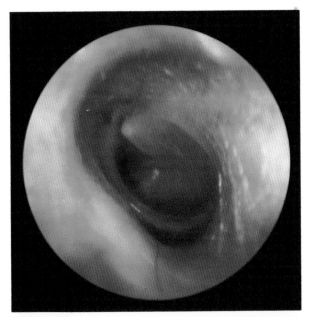

Figure 175

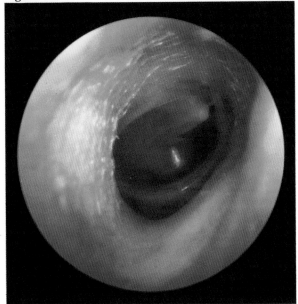

Figure 176

Case Three

John had a history of recurrent tonsillitis and otitis media since the age of 1 year and at 3 years he underwent tonsillectomy and adenoidectomy. Despite this, he continued to have episodes of otitis media.

The appearance of the left eardrum is shown in Figure 177 twelve hours after developing pain in the ear. There is bulging of the upper half of the drum, the outline of the malleus is obscured, and there are prominent blood vessels. One week after treatment with an antibiotic the eardrum returned to normal (Figure 178). Six months later he developed pain in both ears with bulging of the right tympanic membrane, gross inflammation along the handle of the malleus and fluid levels in the lower half of the drum (Figure 179). The left tympanic membrane was erythematous with some distortion of the upper part of the drum (Figure 180).

Four days later there was less inflammation but bubbles were present in both drums indicating effusion in the middle ear cavity (Figures 181 and 182).

Effusion persisted for six weeks but two months after the initial episode both drums returned to normal (Figures 183 and 184).

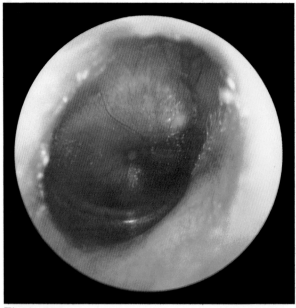

Figure 177

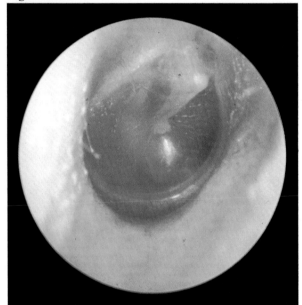

Figure 178

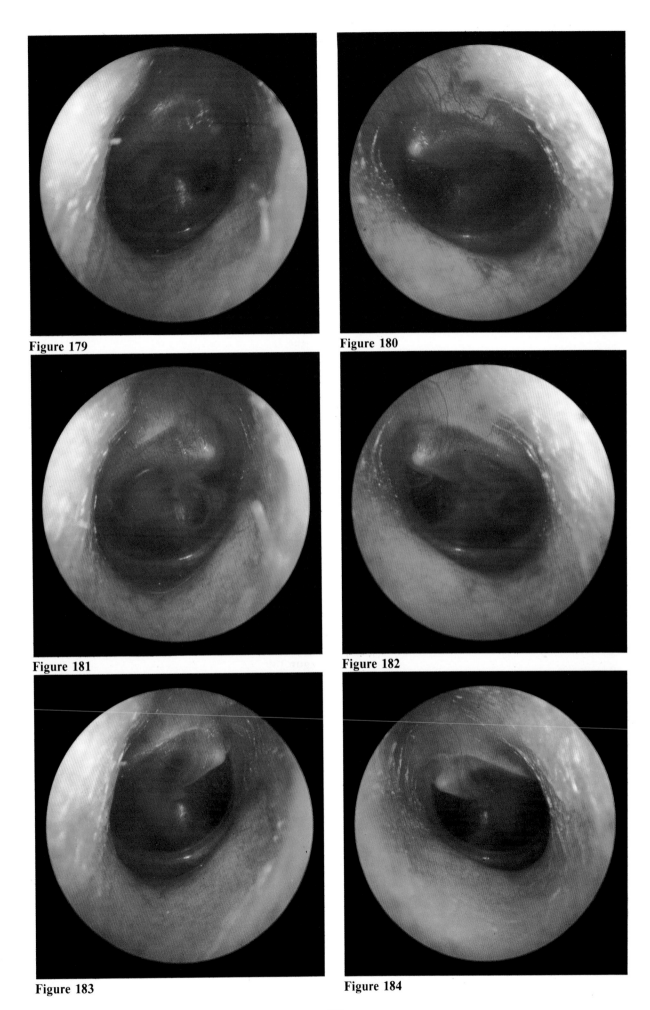

Figure 179

Figure 180

Figure 181

Figure 182

Figure 183

Figure 184

Case Four

Sheila had a longstanding history of upper respiratory tract infection and otitis media since the age of 2.

The distorted left drum with widespread inflammation which was seen during an episode of otitis media when she was aged 4 is shown in Figure 185. Two months later a grommet was inserted in the left tympanic membrane (Figure 186) and in the ensuing six months there was no problem with her ears and her hearing improved. The grommet extruded into the external canal four months after insertion when she suffered a further episode of otitis media (Figure 187). She had another flare-up of acute earache accompanied by inflammation of the left eardrum and fluid in the middle ear four weeks later (Figure 188). Within one week this had partially resolved with antibiotic treatment (Figure 189).

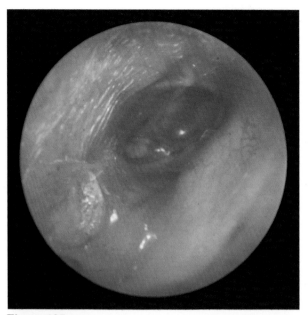

Figure 185

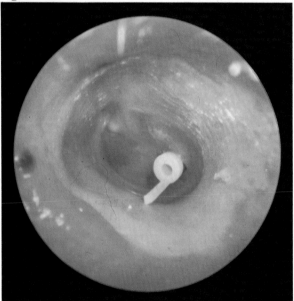

Figure 186

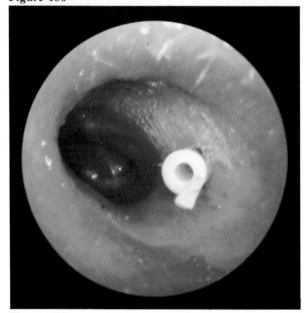

Figure 187

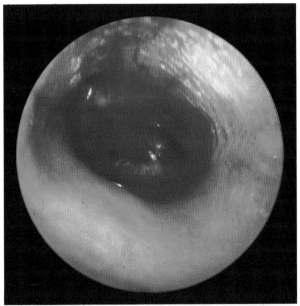

Figure 188

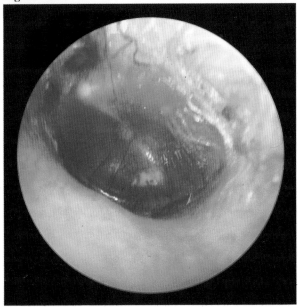

Figure 189

Case Five

Stewart had recurrent upper respiratory tract infections with several episodes of acute otitis media from the age of 1 which responded rapidly to treatment with antibiotics. The appearance of the right ear is shown in Figure 190, 12 hours after the onset of an acute episode of earache when he was aged 3 years. The infection responded rapidly to antibiotics and one week later the appearance was normal (Figure 191).

During a routine examination when he was aged 4 years he was seen to have a symptomless inflammation of the right ear with evidence of fluid behind the drum (Figure 192). Two months later there was a spontaneous return to normal appearances (Figure 193).

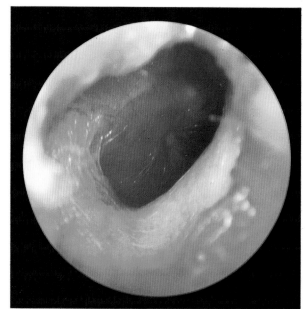

Figure 190

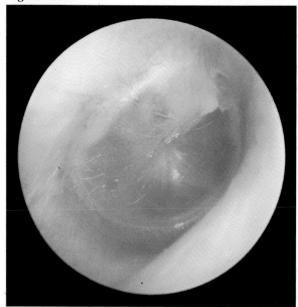

Figure 191

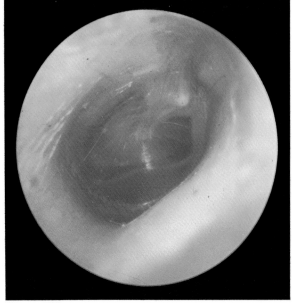

Figure 192

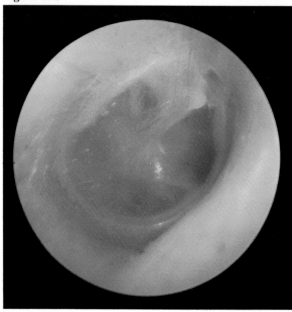

Figure 193

INDEX